GROW
HAIR
IN
12
WEEKS

GROW HAIR
IN
12
WEEKS

The Natural, Healthy Way to Save What
You Have and Restore What You Don't
in Less Than 1 Hour a Week

By

RIQUETTE

with Sallie Batson

Crown Trade Paperbacks/New York

Published by Crown Publishers, Inc.,
201 East 50th Street, New York, New York 10022.
Member of the Crown Publishing Group.

Crown Trade Paperbacks™ and colophon are trademarks of Crown Publishers, Inc.

Manufactured in the United States of America

Library of Congress Cataloging-in-Publication Data
Hofstein, Riquette.
   Grow hair in 12 weeks—the natural, healthy way to save what you have and restore what you don't in less than 1 hour a week.

   1. Hair—Growth.   2. Hair—Care and hygiene.
I. Batson, Sallie.   II. Title.   III. Title: Grow
hair in 12 weeks.
RL91.H67   1988   616.5'46   87-35679

ISBN 0-517-58714-9

10 9 8 7 6 5 4 3 2 1

First Paperback Edition

To my parents, Jacques and Sarah Hofstein, and to my sister, Paulette, for their total love and understanding in allowing me to grow and discover who I really am, without question and with total trust

AUTHOR'S NOTE

All plants, like all medicines, may be dangerous if used improperly. If they are taken internally when prescribed for external use, or if they are taken in excess or over too long a time, allergic reactions and unpredictable sensitivities may develop.

To determine whether you are allergic to any of the recipes in this book, test preparations on a small patch of skin before using them on the hair, scalp or face.

Every effort has been made to ensure that the recipes and substances used in this book are safe when used as directed.

Keep herbs fresh and conditions of use as sterile as possible.

CONTENTS

INTRODUCTION
Meet Riquette

|||||||||||||||||||||||||||||||||||||||||||||||||||||||||||||||||||||||||

Ask this petite dynamo with an electric spray of curls and dazzling, dancing eyes what she does for a living, and Riquette will answer:

"I grow hair on people's heads."

Indeed she does. And what's more, she guarantees it. She also performs this feat without dangerous chemicals or invasive medical or surgical procedures.

"I tell people who do my treatments that I promise—I guarantee—them three things: One, that I can turn their 'peach fuzz' into hair in twelve weeks; two, that I will totally transform the texture of their hair; and, three, that I will stop further hair loss."

There is no conceit in her statement. In the twenty-two years since she began developing her program of totally safe treatments made from simple, natural ingredients, she has grown hair on hundreds of heads. She currently sees more than 750 clients—each of whom came to her as a referral from another client—in her Hollywood clinic.

"Nobody *has* to be bald," Riquette contends. "I have the knowledge, the ability, to stop hair loss without using drugs or chemicals and without surgery. I have used my techniques to save my own hair and to stop hair loss, and I can help you."

Indeed, Riquette uses no drugs, such as the much-touted Minoxidil, or potentially hazardous chemicals, which may cause long-term side effects. "Most of the ingredients I use are herbs and plants, such as basil, rosemary and lemon. Even the pure castile soap, which is made of olive oil and lye, is extremely gentle," she explains, adding that she does nothing to damage the hair further, such as weaving or suturing artificial hair to existing hair or the scalp, nor does she attach wigs or hairpieces with spirit gum or pins.

Riquette's reputation as the gourmet chef of kitchen cosmetics has grown so that she is in great demand as a speaker and lecturer, not to mention as a guest on television.

Whether she is tantalizing TV host David Letterman with the use of carnation oil to attract the opposite sex, massaging her astonishing Slougher Cocktail into the famous bald head of Don Rickles on "The Merv Griffin Show," demonstrating how to make a facial treatment from leftover vegetables at a luncheon workshop for women executives, or teaching a young client how to cure his painfully pimpled skin with carrot juice, Riquette knows what she is doing.

Trained in the European tradition under the strict tutelage of the masters of makeup, hairstyling and skin care, Riquette

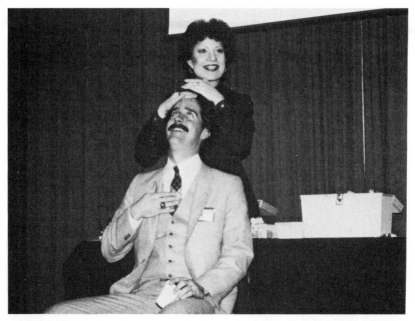

When leading seminars for companies and organizations, Riquette gets the men into the act as well as the women. A volunteer from a workshop for employees at the Cleveland Clinic allows her to demonstrate how her hair rejuvenation program works.

earned advanced degrees and certifications giving her license to work in fourteen countries in Europe and North America. This formal training is augmented by her insatiable curiosity about the body and about beauty, which has caused her to delve into history and nature, not to mention corner markets and her own kitchen cabinets, to experiment and create a wealth of information in this field.

Born in Cairo, Egypt, Riquette moved to Paris as a child with her parents, Jacques and Sarah Hofstein, and her sister, Paulette. At the age of eight, she apprenticed herself to a hair-styling school near the family's new home. Says Riquette, "I believe I started working with hair before I could walk! I *always* knew this was what I wanted to do, so, when we went to

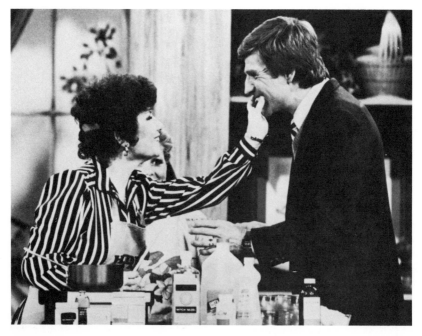

Riquette shows "Hour Magazine" host Gary Collins how men can care for their hair and skin with homemade products such as this Honey and Apricot After Shave she whipped up in a blender.

Paris..." Her Gallic shrug is punctuated by a musical laugh.

Riquette was able to persuade her parents, as well as the headmaster of the school, to let her run errands for the instructors in return for listening to the lectures and watching their demonstrations. "I don't know if they gave in because they thought it was a cute idea and that I would get bored once I found out how hard the work was, or so I would be quiet, but they agreed to let me do it so long as I was in school and kept my grades up."

When Riquette was fourteen, the family moved once more, settling in Sydney, Australia. Riquette, who spoke no English at the time, continued her quest for knowledge, this time beginning a four-year apprenticeship under Alexander of Alex-

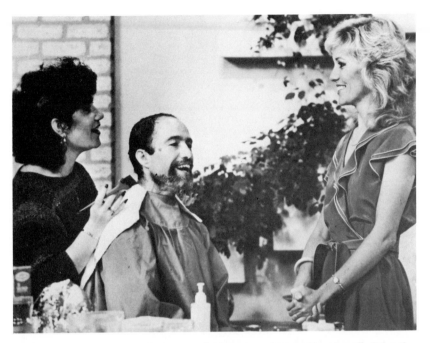

Riquette demonstrates her hair-growth program on "A.M. Los Angeles" for the show's hostess, Ann Martin. The willing model is Eliot Rosen, a client who was so pleased with his results that he was willing to talk about it on camera.

ander International Hairdressers, while she completed high school. "My family...they were just wonderful. Mummy went with me most of the time, helping me get from one school to another. I used her as a model...I used my whole family as models," she laughs.

"My mother's hair has been cut and colored and permed in every way imaginable. I even practiced rolling curls and making waves on my father's head. He had lovely black hair, with a pompadour that he brushed back at the forehead. I can remember him sitting in his chair reading his newspaper while I massaged his scalp and put rollers in his hair—over and over and over again."

Riquette's formal training continued for four more years at

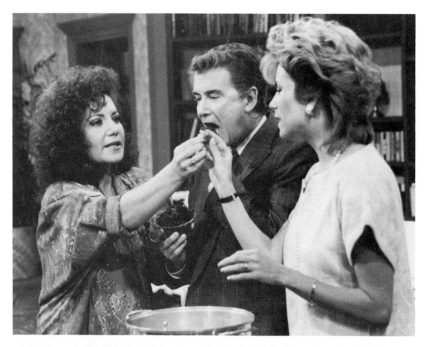

Riquette gets New York's "Morning Show" hosts Regis Philbin and Kathy Lee Gifford to sample parsley, nature's breath freshener, before she tosses it into her versatile vegetable soup that can be eaten or pureed in a blender for hair and face treatments.

the Ultimo Beauty Technical College in Sydney. She then set out to study with the masters in the European beauty capitals of Rome, London, Munich, Paris and Geneva. She returned to Australia armed with awards and degrees from the Schwarz-kopf Institute of Hair Research in Munich, the International College of Aesthetics in Rome, from London's Max Factor Makeup School, and from La Prairie, the famous spa and skin-care institute in Geneva. She holds a certificate in trico-logy—the scientific study of the hair and root—from the René Furterer Institute in Paris. She has also done extensive study in the biochemistry of the hair, scalp and skin, especially with regard to the ingredients in products used in their care.

She was barely twenty when she opened her own salon in Sydney, called Riquette's Place. Since then she has operated ten such head-to-toe beauty clinics, in Europe and the Far East as well as Australia and the United States.

Ever interested in the performing arts, Riquette also saw the potential for work as a makeup artist and hairstylist in Australia's then-budding film and television industry. "I started doing hair and makeup for commercials and photo shoots, then for television and movies," she explains.

During this period of both personal and professional growth, Riquette expanded her work as a free-lance makeup artist in films and TV, and developed a reputation as an image consultant. Expanding her credentials, she received accreditation from Revlon International.

She also expanded her personal research inward. "I had begun to concentrate on my study of the skin in hopes of clearing up my own problems," Riquette confides. "When I was a teenager I had horrible, horrible acne. It was so bad at times that all you could see was my eyes. Nothing done by doctors, or anyone else I consulted, helped very much."

Following her instincts, Riquette called upon her training and investigated the possibilities of nutritional care, altering her diet and taking vitamin supplements, along with a carefully planned program of skin treatments. This involved cleansing, toning and moisturizing her sensitive skin with herbal compounds that both calmed the irritation and treated the causes of her skin allergies and acne.

She began to treat her hair similarly. "It was very fragile, bushy with tight curls. I couldn't get a comb through it, it was so curly. I straightened it, which was no problem for a while, but the chemicals I used on my hair caused terrible damage. My hair broke at a touch and then it began to fall out."

Once again, Riquette turned to common sense—diet and nutrition—and nature for help. "I knew that through the ages people had used herbs, roots and leaves to treat their hair and make it healthy and beautiful. I began to research what these plants were and how they were used. Then I studied my hair and its root under a microscope to determine exactly what was wrong with it, as I was taught in tricology. Finally I experimented with herbs and plants that were known to be good for the problems I diagnosed, trying one thing and then another until I came upon the right combination—or combinations—that could correct these problems. As a result, I transformed my hair to what it is today—lush, manageable and healthy."

By the time she had saved her own hair, Riquette had devised a complete program of scalp and hair treatments that actually curb hair loss and promote growth, now called Riquette's Hair Rejuvenation Program.

By the mid-1970s, Riquette's work brought her to the attention of Walt Disney Productions, which was then producing a big adventure film, *Ride the Wild Pony,* that would be shooting in the Australian outback.

Soon she was out in the bush, far from metropolitan Sydney, hard at work on the film. "I had actors and actresses sitting on an upturned apple crate while I did their hair," she laughs. "I even had to create a hairstyle for a pony."

It was in 1975, when she came to the United States for the premiere of *Ride the Wild Pony,* that Riquette decided to move to this country. "I came here for six weeks," she reminisces, "and decided to stay."

Later that year she opened her first Riquette's Place in New York.

Riquette moved her base of operations to Cleveland, Ohio, where she opened eight complete Riquette's Place beauty clinics and a school. Since 1982 she has been headquartered in Hollywood, where her Riquette International Clinic caters to the hair and skin-care needs of a select clientele from the worlds of entertainment and business.

Wherever she has worked, Riquette's ability to stop hair loss and turn "peach fuzz" into hair, as well as her entertaining, uncanny knack for turning ordinary things that you would find in an everyday kitchen into extraordinary beauty products, have made her in demand as a speaker.

Riquette's reputation as an image consultant has been extended into the boardrooms of such corporations as General Motors, Stouffer's and the Cleveland Clinic, as well as modeling agencies, civic and community service clubs and such internationally known fashion and cosmetic houses as Christian Dior.

Recently, Riquette has noticed a marked increase in the number of people—almost as many women as men—coming to her especially to stop hair loss. This awareness has prompted her to write this book.

Read on. Riquette is an able teacher and motivator who truly believes that it's never too late to have a beautiful head of hair.

Sallie Batson

GROW HAIR IN 12 WEEKS

1

ANYONE CAN HAVE A WONDERFUL HEAD OF HAIR

||||||||||||||||||||||||||||||||||||||||||||||||||||||||||||||||||||||||||||

At birth, each of us had the *potential* to have a lifetime of healthy, beautiful hair. Sadly, this potential has never been fulfilled by many of us.

To understand what this means and to put everything back on track so that anyone can attain the wonderful head of hair each one of us is meant to have, we must talk a bit about hair, and then about how things got out of hand.

WHAT IS HAIR?

Hair is *pilus*, a slender, threadlike fiber on the body. It is a protein—97 percent protein, in fact—with the remaining 3 percent made up of amino acids, minerals and other trace elements.

We have hair of various types all over our bodies. In fact, the only places we *don't* have some form of hair are the soles of our feet, the palms of our hands and our lips. The hair that grows on our heads is quite possibly the most decorative feature of—or on—the human body. While it provides insulation for our heads, protecting it from heat and cold, it also has definite ornamental purposes.

We are often described in terms of our hair: "Isn't she a lovely redhead?" "Frank is so distinguished, with that gray hair at his temples." "The tall, blond lifeguard..." "The white-haired gentleman in the navy pinstriped suit..." "The bald guy..."

The hair we will be discussing in these pages is the hair on our heads... or at least the hair we *want* to have on our heads. I contend that a healthy head of hair is our birthright, and it's time we all stepped up to claim it!

Hair has three distinct layers. The *cuticle*, or exterior layer, is composed of overlapping "shingles," flat, transparent pieces that protect the inner parts of the hair shaft. The *cortex*, the second layer, is made up of elongated cells that grow end on end rather than overlapping and give the hair its flexibility and tensile strength. The cortex contains the pigments that give our hair its natural color; when hair turns gray, this source of pigmentation has been depleted. The innermost layer of the hair is the *medulla*. It is composed of two rows of cells that grow side by side through the length of the shaft. It determines the strength, body and elasticity of the hair.

When any one of these layers is damaged, the hair is weak-

Hair Shaft

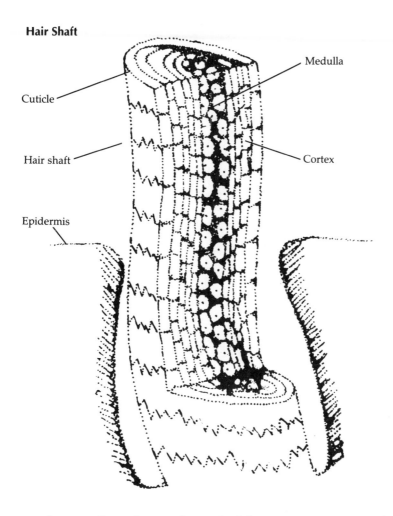

Cuticle

Medulla

Hair shaft

Cortex

Epidermis

ened, sometimes beyond repair. My treatments not only halt such damage but repair it as well.

There are an estimated one thousand hairs per square inch on the average scalp, which amounts to as many as 140,000 hairs per head.

I tell my clients to think of their hair as a green onion. The root, which grows under the scalp, is the living part, while the

How Hair Grows

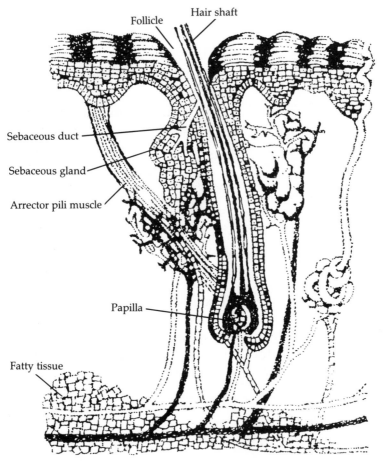

hair shaft—the green part of the onion—which is on the out-side, is not living.

Each hair grows from a root, the *papilla*, which is alive. This root is nourished by the bloodstream, making circulation through the scalp essential to healthy hair. When the root is healthy, the hair grows with ease; when it is unhealthy, the hair reflects this as well. In the next chapter I will introduce you to your own root so that you will have a clearer picture of the condition of your hair and scalp.

HOW DOES HAIR GROW?

Hair grows at a rate of approximately one-half inch per month from two to six years, then rests for about three months before being pushed out by a new hair that has been slowly growing its way up through the skin. On the average, if both the hair and its root as well as the scalp, with its intricate network of nerves and sebaceous (oil) glands, are in working order, this "life" lasts about four years.

When the cycle is normal, we lose eighty to one hundred hairs per day. If, when you run your fingers through your hair, it comes out easily, the hair was most probably ready to be released by the papilla so that a new hair could begin to grow. If your loss is light—within that range of eighty to one hundred hairs per day—your hair and scalp are normal and you should have nothing to worry about.

If, when you pull your fingers through your hair, you come out with a handful, you have a hair-loss problem, just as you would if you were to see a lot of hair in the basin or tub after washing your hair. Such massive hair loss is *not* natural, even if your father is bald.

If you are *not* shedding, your roots are not producing new hair. The formation of new growth depends entirely upon how much nourishment each papilla and root get from the bloodstream, and how clean the scalp is, so that new hair can push its way through to the surface.

The scalp, by the way, is the hardest place on our bodies for blood to reach. Like our fingertips and toes, it is an extremity. The treatments you will learn from me in this book are designed to stimulate blood flow to the scalp to encourage hair growth.

WHY DO WE LOSE HAIR?

In the twenty-two years I have been working and studying hair loss, I have found that 99 percent of all hair loss in men and in women is caused by one thing—excessive oil. This oil, called *sebum*, clogs the pores of the scalp and stifles follicle growth. In time, the root is asphyxiated, making it impossible for new hair to grow.

This loss is manifested in various ways, most commonly as a receding hairline; hereditary male pattern baldness (MPB), which is properly known as *androgenetic alopecia*, is a condition afflicting *approximately half* of the male population by the age of fifty, and is the cause of the overall thinning most often experienced by women. Another form of hair loss in women, *alopecia areata*, is the sudden balding in irregular patches on the scalp. In most of these cases, the nervous system has been injured in some way, causing the affected area to be poorly nourished.

Hair loss is, according to geneticists, a secondary sexual characteristic of males, influenced by hormones as well as the positioning of the hair on the head. Women don't have the same hormonal structure as men, and our hair grows differently—at an angle and with the follicles set deeper into the scalp.

The follicles on top of a man's head grow straight up; consequently, when oil is released from the scalp, it has no place to go. On a woman's head, it can slip down the hair shaft toward the end; on a man's, it can only slide back to where it came from—the scalp.

If the scalp is not cleaned properly, this oil becomes wax, clogging the pores. When a hair is shed, its successor cannot come out. It becomes weak and literally goes to sleep under the scalp. The few hairs that manage to push through that waxy barrier are so puny that they are ready to fall out as soon as they break through.

Such are the circumstances leading to MPB.

**Examples of Male
Pattern Baldness**

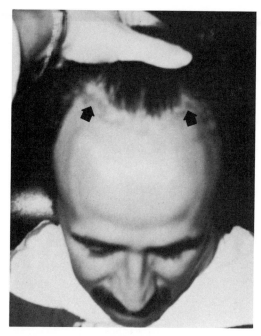

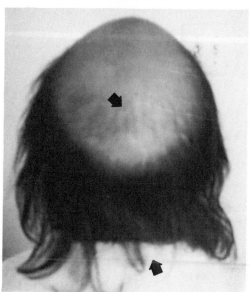

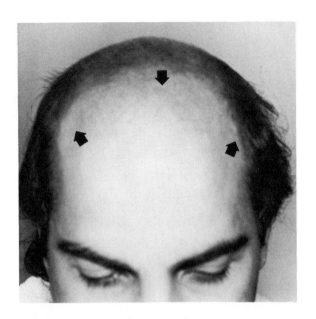

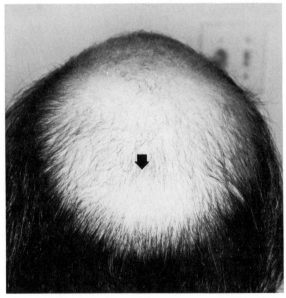

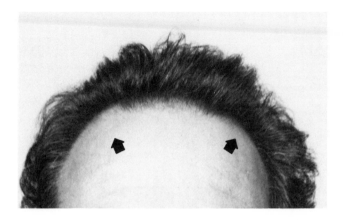

This is what it looks like.

It *can* be stopped.

When I unclog the pores on the scalp, and the dormant hair sees the light of day, it grows in healthy and strong, if given proper care. Rub your fingers across your scalp. If you can feel fuzz, there is a very good possibility that you can turn it into hair with my twelve-week treatment program.

ALL IN THE FAMILY?

Balding is *not* hereditary, but the *tendency* toward balding—or baldness—is. You can choose to not go bald by following my advice rather than in your parents' footsteps, and it is never too late to take that first step.

Here's what one of my clients told me not long after he had completed the initial Twelve-Week Hair Rejuvenation Program:

"Both of my grandfathers, as well as my father, were 80 percent bald by their mid-twenties," according to Sandor Black, an actor and musician. "I came to you to see if we could alleviate the inevitability of this happening to me."

When Sandor started the treatments, he had such weak hair that it definitely would have fallen out had he not begun the program. He was referred to me, as are all my clients, by a friend who was so excited about the changes—and especially the growth—in his own hair that he wanted *everyone* to know about me and how I stopped him from going bald.

Sandor says that he is truly grateful to this good friend. "I am very happy to say that after just four months of treatments, I see genuine new hair growth and an undeniable difference in the texture and look of my hair as well as a continuing full head of hair at twenty-seven years old."

A brother and sister I know are prime examples of the role genetics plays with regard to the condition and type of hair we have, even though they initially appear to have very different hair. David and Lydia Finzi both have fine hair that is oily at the roots and very dry at the ends.

Sister and brother Lydia and David Finzi have very similar hair. Both have fine hair that is oily at the roots and very dry on the ends.

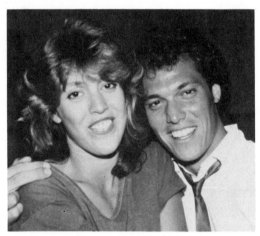

David's hair had begun to thin out considerably through the crown. His hairline was receding drastically on both sides in front. His forehead was shiny and his scalp very oily, which made his hair quite stringy. His scalp was very itchy and his severe dandruff made it impossible for him to wear dark colors.

Before

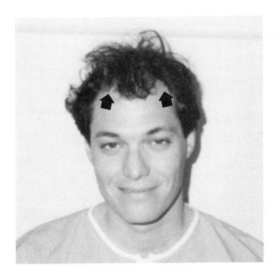

After

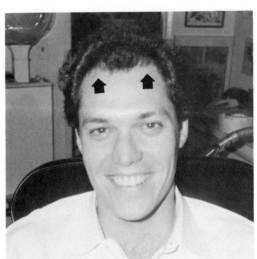

Lydia's hair, though not as curly as her brother's, was also very oily at the roots and extremely dry—almost brittle—at the ends. Although she had her hair professionally colored

Before

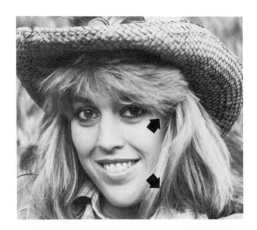

After

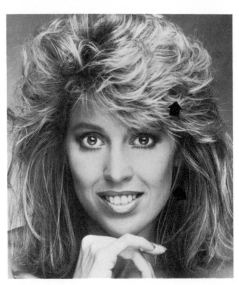

and cut, she was plagued by its dull tone and lack of sheen. Lydia began the treatments to restore health to her thinning hair.

Upon seeing the improvement in his younger sister's hair, David wanted to know what I could do for him. He was intrigued with what Lydia had told him about how I stopped balding. In only three weeks of treatments, David began to sprout hair where I could neither feel nor see peach fuzz! His oiliness is under control, and his hair no longer coils in greasy curls across his forehead.

HAIR TELLS TALES

Your hair has a way of telling you if your body is in balance.

If you are healthy—physically as well as emotionally—your hair will be radiant and shining and your scalp pliant and moist.

If you are not well physically, or if you are upset emotionally, your hair becomes dull and lifeless—it will begin to fall out, and your scalp will become waxy with the overproduction of your traumatized sebaceous glands.

Truly, any major changes in our lives can be reflected in the condition of our hair, scalp and skin. If we are well and happy, we reflect this health and well-being in the condition of our hair and scalp. If we are in a slump, that slump is often manifested in the appearance of our hair and scalp.

Rumors to the contrary, there is little concrete medical evidence that stress—regardless of its origin—actually contributes to balding. It just seems that way.

The truth is that when we are under stress, we let our basic health habits go. Think about it:

You are pushing a deadline for a major project at work. Your boss has as much as told you that your job is on the line. How do you react?

First of all, you start drinking more coffee and soft drinks than usual, and if you're still a smoker, you start smoking more than ever. By doing this, you increase the poisons from caffeine and nicotine in your body, taking in far larger quantities than when you are not under such pressure.

Then you work until all hours, racing into the office without breakfast in the morning. You pick up coffee and a sweet roll, which you gobble at your desk, and if you eat lunch at all, you gulp down fast food from the deli downstairs. You might unwind at the bar down the block, wash down the free hors d'oeuvres and salted nuts with a couple of drinks. Dinner may be take-out Chinese or fried chicken, eaten as you hunch over your papers to be ready to start the process all over again the following day.

You get no exercise, other than racing from place to place, and you sleep irregular hours. More than likely, you don't pay a lot of attention to your face: you touch it with inkstained hands; you run your fingers through your hair and then rest your chin in your hand, transferring the oils and dirt from one to the other. You give your hair a quick washing, paying little attention to conditioning or rinsing, if you wash it at all. In no time at all, your skin becomes sallow and sensitive. Your hair becomes dull and lifeless, and before you know it, it is falling out in bunches. This is not caused directly by stress, but by what you have done to your body while you are under stress.

Your hair is one of the first places your body shows distress. Illness, medication and imbalances in nutrition all show up in your hair and scalp, as well as in your skin. Even aspirin and over-the-counter allergy pills or cold tablets can have a negative effect on your hair, especially if your hair is chemically treated with color or a permanent.

FOOD FOR THOUGHT

Just as the residue from drugs and medications and all the other negative things that we put in our bodies show up in our hair, the *positive* results of nutritional care are evidenced there also. There are no pills we can take or miracle foods we can eat to have healthy hair, but we *can* feed our hair and scalp by eating the foods that promote physical health and well-being.

Without going into any medical or chemical explanations, I want you to take a candid look at your daily diet. Do you eat a lot of red meat? Fried foods? White breads and processed sugars? Butter? Do you drink a lot of coffee, tea or caffeine-laden colas? Alcohol? Candy? If you do, you are selling your body—and your hair—short.

Start by rethinking your approach to food. One of the most helpful bits of advice I can give you is to reverse your eating habits. Make breakfast the main meal of your day. As the old saying goes: In the morning, eat like a queen, at lunchtime, eat like a princess, and at night, eat like a pauper. Have most of your daily food intake in the morning, when you will have longer to digest it before going to bed. Your body will work much more efficiently this way!

The health of the hair, according to Dr. Benjamin Colimore, a nutrition consultant specializing in homeopathy, is "not contingent on any one factor to do the entire job. There is only the high quality, sufficient quantity and proper balance of *all* nutrients and the efficiency of the body's enzyme systems to balance the condition of the root and scalp."

Just as balance is the key to the success of the treatments I put *on* the hair and scalp, balance is essential to nutrition, which is essential to the body's health, which in turn is essential to a healthy head of hair. See how everything is related?

Dr. Colimore uses my Hair Rejuvenation Program to enhance his own hair and scalp, and follows his own advice about diet and nutrition. He stresses that we must achieve a balance among the essential nutrients, protein, fat and carbohydrates, as well as vitamins and minerals, to achieve a healthy, balanced body.

We need to eat a variety of foods in each of these groups for maximum health. Only one-fifth of our daily protein intake should come from meats, including fish and fowl. Everything I have read or been told points to the elimination of red meats from our diet. It would be unrealistic for me to tell you to stop eating beef or your hair won't grow, so I will resist that temptation. Instead, I will caution you to limit your red meat intake to once a week.

Foods rich in the B vitamins (leafy green vegetables, whole grains, liver, peas and beans, fish, cheese and eggs), vitamin A (spinach, kale, broccoli, sweet potatoes, beets, chicory, watercress, collard greens, tomatoes, parsnips, watercress, butternut squash, cantaloupes and papayas) and vitamin C (citrus fruits such as oranges and grapefruits, as well as potatoes, tomatoes, melons, strawberries, cauliflower, sweet peppers and green vegetables like broccoli, kale and cabbage) are vital to the health and well-being of your hair and scalp, as are calcium-rich foods such as canned fish (bones and all), fortified milk, cheese, tofu, yogurt, oysters and kidney beans.

Calf and beef liver, dried beans, peas, shrimp, oysters and other seafoods, prunes, whole wheat, most nuts and fruits and many other unprocessed foods will provide the copper that is helpful in creating healthy hair, while these mineral-rich foods plus asparagus, egg yolks, poultry, molasses, soybean flower, oatmeal, leafy green vegetables, dried peaches, raisins and red meat provide the iron needed by the body.

Other minerals that contribute to full, rich hair are zinc (in poultry, nuts, seeds, legumes, eggs, whole grains, dry milk, wheat germ, brewer's yeast and ground mustard), iodine (in seafood, iodized and sea salts, kelp and other seaweeds, onions and vegetables grown in iron-rich soil) and sulfur (in eggs, fish, garlic, onions, dried beans, cabbage and asparagus).

Avoid foods that are high in oils and fats—red meats, fried foods, most nuts and nut products—and limit your intake of shellfish and iodized salt because they contain *too much* iodine. Iodine does help hair growth, but too much can cause acne.

Chocolate and cocoa products, cheese, sugars, caffeine-laden soft drinks, coffee and tea, as well as alcohol, should be eliminated or at least restricted, because they can trigger systemic problems that upset the delicate balance between your hair and its environment, the scalp.

The chemical content of the hair is so drastically altered by pollutants that the real nutritional effects of the diet can be lost unless we can reach and maintain that wonderful, delicate balance.

THE FINE ART OF BRUSHING

What we do to our hair is as damaging as what we *don't* do. Throughout this book I will call your attention to the ways that we assault our hair and scalp with blow dryers, chemical processing and environmental pollutants, to make you aware of these conditions.

The treatments in the basic Hair Rejuvenation Program have been designed with attention to the hair's physical needs. They will rectify situations that promote further damage.

Before you begin treating your hair, you will need to prepare it by brushing it completely and thoroughly to loosen dust, dead cells and pollution from both hair and scalp and increase blood circulation in the scalp.

Do not use just any hairbrush. Buy a good natural-bristle brush, because these bristles are pliant and won't damage your hair. Look for a brush that is firm, yet has flexible bristles that give a little as you move them through your hair. Two readily available brand-name brushes are by Mason and Pearson, which makes both natural bristle and combination plastic and natural bristle models with bristles embedded in a flexible rubber base on a solid, easy-to-hold handle, and by Denman, which offers a brush with smooth, rubbery teeth in a supple rubber head. The bristles should be rounded, not sharp and pointed.

Purchase a good comb, too. It should have rounded teeth with no rough edges. Texture of the teeth, whether it is fine-toothed or full, should depend upon your hair type.

Every member of your family should have both a brush and

a comb of his or her own. Do not share. You wouldn't dream of sharing toothbrushes—don't share hairbrushes.

Before you put your brush to your hair, I want you to take a good look at it. This is serious business. When was the last time you washed it? And your comb? And what about the ones stashed in your attaché case or desk? Unless they are brand-new, my guess is that you can't remember. Am I right?

When I see people's brushes and combs beside their sinks, I become ill at the very sight of them. Now, I am not talking about people who don't know better. These are friends who dress immaculately, who wouldn't think of putting their dirty clothes back on after taking a bath.

Would you believe that they think nothing of washing their hair and then combing it out with a comb that hasn't been washed in months? Then they blow-dry their hair with a brush that is just as dirty!

For beautiful, healthy hair, *wash your brush and comb every time you wash your hair.*

Every time.

Without fail.

I am quite serious about this. Cultivate the habit of taking them into the shower with you and cleaning them when you wash your scalp and hair. It won't take more than a minute!

To clean your comb and brush, comb hair out of the dry brush, then squirt a small amount of shampoo (pages 88–89) into the head of the brush. Run your comb through the bristles of the brush as you dip it into your bath water or dampen it a bit under the shower. Shampoo is an excellent cleaning product for your brushes and combs because it is created to dissolve the waxes and oils found in the hair and produced by the scalp. Rinse thoroughly under hot water and repeat the washing process. Shake out the excess water and dry your brush and comb on a terry towel.

If my warnings about cleanliness do not inspire you to cultivate this practice, here is another important reason to use clean tools: A clean brush and comb will enable you actually to see the amount of hair that comes out on a day-to-day basis. You have probably become so accustomed to seeing a brush full of hair that this procedure will allow you to see how little hair comes out as you follow the treatments of this program.

To brush your hair, use your new natural-bristle brush and lean forward at the waist for added scalp stimulation. Brush first from the neck forward to your forehead, and then from the sides to the top of your head. Finally, brush from the forehead back toward the neck.

If your hair is long and tangled, work to unsnarl these tangles from the ends, at the tangles, up the length of the hair to the scalp. Brush gently without pulling on your hair or irritating your scalp.

Grooming, nutrition, physical well-being—these are all part of having the shining, luxuriant hair you are entitled to.

2

GETTING TO THE ROOT OF YOUR PROBLEM

Healthy Hair Starts with a Healthy Root

||||||||||||||||||||||||||||||||||||||||||||||||||||||||||||||||||||||||||||||||||||

I learn a great deal about a client from looking at the roots of his or her hair. I can tell if a person has a healthy, balanced diet, or if he eats a lot of red meats and fried foods. I can see if she works around chemicals or in a heavily polluted area, or if he spends a lot of time in the sun or cold. Every root provides vast insight into the state of the person to whom it belongs. Sometimes the story it tells is quite different from that of its owner.

I go to the root of the problem, literally, assessing the condition of the root to determine what needs to be done to repair the situation. I want you to get to know your root so that you can analyze it. This will enable you to understand and subsequently take care of your hair and scalp so that new, healthy hair will grow. Pay attention to what you see and feel. I am going to teach your fingers to "see" what your eyes cannot, even up close.

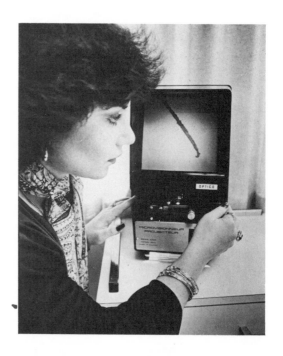

In my clinic, I use a special microscope to examine my clients' hair. This way, I can tell exactly the condition of the root and hair shaft. The hair shown here has an oily root and a weak, dry hair shaft—notice how it is thinner just before the root than elsewhere. The hair is also somewhat damaged, as you can see by the irregular cuticle, or outside layer. My analysis of this hair is that it has an oily root and dry shaft. (Reprinted by permission of the *Akron Beacon Journal*)

In my clinic, I use a special electronic microscope to examine my clients' hair. You can use a simple magnifying glass to see enough of your hair follicle and root to determine its condition.

Pull a hair from your head—from the crown or the front—and look at the end. You should be able to see a little "knot"—that is the bulb or root that fits around the papilla as the hair shaft grows.

If this knot or root is bulb-shaped, like a cotton swab, and is twice the size of the hair shaft, it is a normal root. Such a root is capable of generating normal, healthy hair growth.

**Normal, Balanced,
Healthy Root and Shaft**

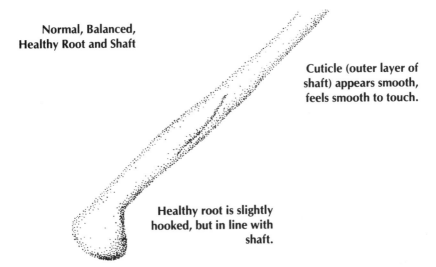

**Cuticle (outer layer of
shaft) appears smooth,
feels smooth to touch.**

**Healthy root is slightly
hooked, but in line with
shaft.**

If this knot is as small as, or smaller than, the hair shaft, or if it ends in a point, the root is weak, if not dead. Check other parts of your head to determine whether the weakness was just in that one hair or whether it appears everywhere.

**Weak hair shaft shows
oil deposited at root,
which curves.**

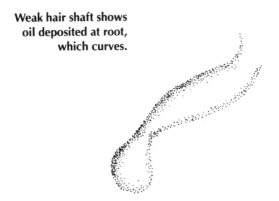

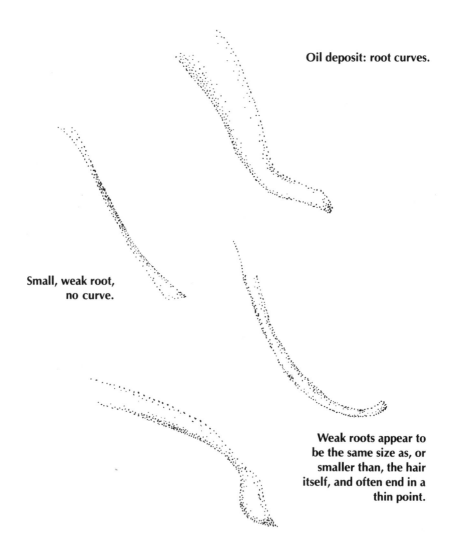

Oil deposit: root curves.

Small, weak root, no curve.

Weak roots appear to be the same size as, or smaller than, the hair itself, and often end in a thin point.

An oily root, indicating an oily scalp, appears jellylike and transparent, as if the end of your hair had been dipped in clear nail polish. You will not be able to see or feel a knot.

Dry scalp is indicated if the knot is dried out. You will probably be able to feel it with your fingertip or nail, but not see it. If your hair breaks off at the scalp, you have serious drying and weakness problems.

You will need plenty of light to be able to see your root. Hold the hair up to a light and study it carefully through a magnifying glass. It will take practice, but you will, in time, learn to recognize what you are seeing.

Take a sample of your hair before you begin treatments, and then repeat this process every three weeks. Tape each strand (across the middle of the shaft, so you won't destroy the root) to your Root Record Chart (pages 26–28). Write down the date that you examined the hair and note your observations about the condition of your hair and scalp. Does your hair feel oily to the touch? Is it dry? Describe the condition and feel of the ends. What does the scalp feel like? What does it look like?

This process will educate you about your root and hair, as well as show how much progress is being made. You will actually be able to see your root improve as your peach fuzz becomes hair; your hair texture is changed, and any abnormal hair loss is stopped.

If you do not see a root on the first hair you pull from your crown, remove another hair in case you broke the first one off at the scalp. If you still fail to detect a root, you have a *very* oily root, even if your hair is very dry.

You can have an oily root and dry hair; in fact, most people do. Most of my clients who complain about a dry scalp really have an oily scalp and root that has been mistreated.

According to the *Journal of the American Medical Association*, 12 percent of males begin losing hair by age 25, 37 percent by age 35. Recent studies also show that roughly 25 percent of women between the ages of 25 and 54 suffer severe thinning of their hair. Of this loss, I find that 99 percent is solely attributable to excess oil in the scalp. That is why I *insist* that you get to know your root!

ROOT RECORD CHART

WEEK 1   DATE:

NOTES:

WEEK 3   DATE:

NOTES:

WEEK 6   DATE:

NOTES:

WEEK 9   DATE:

NOTES:

WEEK 12   DATE:

NOTES:

3

WHO SAID IT COULDN'T BE DONE?

Certainly Not These Believers

||||||||||||||||||||||||||||||||||||||||||||||||||||||||||||||||||||||||||||

What better proof is there that I can do what I promise than photographic documentation of my clients as they go through the series of scalp and hair treatments I give them? These pictures and letters are just a fraction of the success stories I have on record to substantiate the results of this program. What you see are, for the most part, snapshots taken in my clinic so that we might have an accurate record of each client's progress before and during the course of the treatments. As you can tell, I am not a photographer, but even with my lack of skill in that area, you can see the changes that have taken place!

29

TOM LEIGH

I met Tom Leigh when I went into his printing shop to order business cards for the opening of my clinic in Hollywood. When I told him what I do, he became my first client and he has been with me ever since. Before the treatments, there was no hair on his crown, only a light fuzz. His hair was fine, but the curl was wiry and tight. Twelve weeks after he began the treatments, Tom's hair was beginning to fill in through the

Before

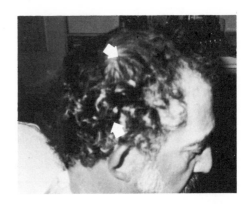

After

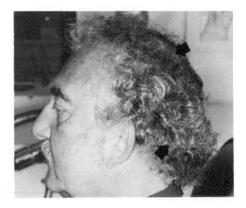

crown, and his hair texture had improved so much that the curl had begun to relax. Today it is soft and full.

Tom continues to have maintenance treatments monthly, and uses the shampoos and rinse I have prescribed for him.

MARIO GOTTUSO

Mario Gottuso is one of my biggest fans! He has referred many of his friends to me, and after almost five years he continues on maintenance treatments to keep his hair and scalp healthy. I have almost become part of his family, watching his daughter grow. I even gave her her first haircut!

Here are two letters that Mario sent to me—one after he completed his initial twelve-week program, and the other four years later.

March 28, 1983

Dear Riquette,

As you know, I was very hesitant about coming to you for hair treatments. Although my hair has been thinning for quite some time, I just didn't believe in any hair-growth programs. I believed that all hair loss was due to heredity.

After watching one of your television spots, I was still unconvinced. My wife, Robin, decided to give you a call for more details.

Robin convinced me to go at least for a consultation. We found you to be very professional and very easy to get along with. Your enthusiasm excited us. You didn't make any unrealistic promises. After looking at my hair under the microscope and seeing how oily the roots were and lis-

tening to your explanation for the treatments, we agreed to begin the twelve-week program.

Needless to say, we began seeing results. It was very obvious after about six weeks that hair was beginning to grow. My scalp was cleaner, and my dandruff was disappearing soon after using the special formula shampoos.

After twelve weeks my hair had shown considerable improvement. We continued for an additional six weeks because we were so pleased with the results.

Robin and I are convinced that my hair growth and quality will continue to improve. My skepticism has turned to belief.

Thank you for your hair treatments and friendship. Your concern for us during our eighteen-week association has been of equal or more value.

Sincerely,

Mario Gottuso, Jr.

April 5, 1987

Dear Riquette,

It has been about four and one half years since I began receiving treatments from you to help control my hair loss. Over the course of time, I and others have noticed that my hair is stronger and that there has been new hair growth.

While I don't ever expect to have my hair fully restored, I am convinced that your hair treatments do work. I have always appreciated the fact that the treatments and shampoos are natural and do not make outlandish claims. Merely keeping my scalp clean through the shampoos and your hair/scalp treatments, which also help drain excessive oil, has helped considerably in allowing for new hair

Before

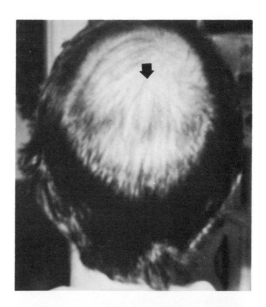

After

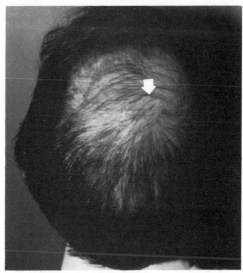

growth and the lessening of hair thinning. If I had started using your program when my hair first started thinning, I would probably still have a full head of hair!

As you recall, I was very skeptical when I came for my first appointment. After diagnosing my problem you recommended a twelve-week program. I seriously doubted that new hair would begin to grow during that time. After about six weeks it was obvious that new hair was growing. I no longer doubted your program. During the course of time, I have switched back to my previous products with miserable results. My hair became weak, dandruff reappeared, and my scalp became excessively oily again. Your products and program do work.

I have appreciated your open and honest manner. While you might encourage me to increase my maintenance program from the treatments every two months to encourage more hair growth, you have never tried to force any products for me to use. You allow me to follow my own program under your direction. You also never promised more than you could deliver. The results I have had with my hair are exactly what you said would happen.

It is a long drive to come in for treatments, but well worth it. My hair is stronger and new hair continues to grow. More important, the friendship my family and I have developed with you make the trips even more worthwhile.

Sincerely,

Mario Gottuso, Jr.

RICK RISO

Entertainer and recording artist Rick Riso started visibly losing his hair in his mid-twenties, a situation that was critical by the time he was thirty-four. A talented writer, singer and lead guitarist, Rick rarely smiled, even for his publicity pictures. By the time he started coming to me, he was hiding behind a full beard and mustache and darkly tinted glasses.

Before

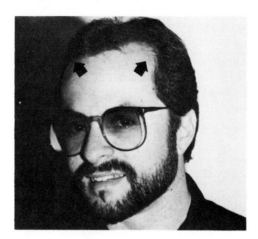

After

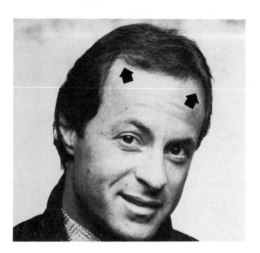

In three months, he had noticeable regrowth around his hairline, and the shiny waxiness and pimples across his forehead were almost gone. The texture of his hair had changed from oily, wiry and lifeless to beautifully balanced, shining and healthy. Rick felt so much better about his appearance that he had a new set of photographs taken. You can see from these pictures how much improvement there has been. Notice how much more self-assured he appears, and how much better his skin looks.

In the three years since Rick began my treatments, he continues to show improvement. His hair loss has stopped so that there is no more than the average loss of hair that is ready to fall out. More important, the hair that grew back has remained. Rick's skin is more supple, with fewer wrinkles at thirty-seven than he had at thirty-three!

DARBY SWITZER

When Darby heard I was writing a book, he rushed to send this wonderful tribute to me:

> As a cameraman, my world is composed primarily of visual elements. The success of my career depends on my ability to interpret and present these components in an attractive manner. Due to this emphasis on appearance, my clients, initially, may judge my competence as an image-maker by the image that I personally reflect. Although hair loss is not an indication of poor grooming, I feel that in my case it detracted from my overall appearance.
>
> In 1982, while shooting a story about Riquette, I learned of her unique hair-growth program. At this time I was losing my hair at an alarming rate. Convinced that I would be bald within a year or two, I was anxious to learn more about her approach to this problem. Reasoning that I had nothing to lose but my hair, I gladly started the recommended treatments. Within a few months, I could see the

results. The rate of hair loss slowed and I actually began to see new hair. Now, after five years, the hair loss has almost completely stopped and a new hairline has emerged. I am very pleased with Riquette's program and highly recommend it.

Before

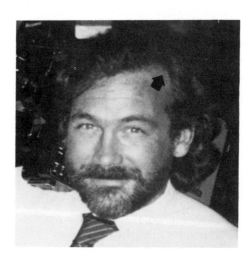

After

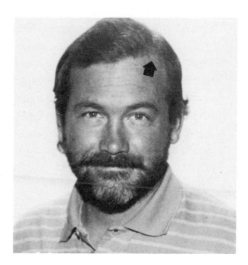

Darby's words and photographs tell it all. His hairline is stronger and healthier than ever before, and his oily, waxy scalp condition has cleared up!

DANIEL E. URENDA

April 6, 1983

Riquette:

I have to confess that I had reservations at first, but that changed after my first consultation with you. I became aware that not only are you a professional in your field, but that you are genuinely concerned and interested in helping people. Your treatments have helped rejuvenate my hair.

Now, after several treatments, I can testify that your treatments do work. My hair is naturally darker and more manageable than ever, and I have less loss of hair. This is all a result of feeding my scalp what it was missing by the use of your products and treatments.

Your personal attention and advice on my hair needs are well worth my time. I would encourage all who are contemplating doing something positive for themselves to see you. They have nothing to lose and a healthy outlook to gain.

Sincerely,

Daniel E. Urenda

Daniel had classic male pattern baldness—the circular loss at the crown and the receding hairline. I found this unusual because he is Mexican, and Mexicans are not known for hair loss. On the contrary, they usually have excellent hair and are rarely bald.

Before

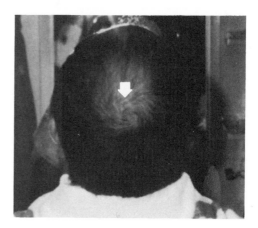

After

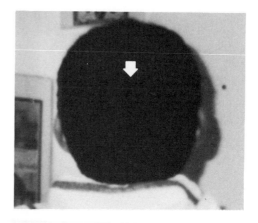

Daniel, as you can see by his pictures, has had wonderful results from the treatments.

ARLENE ABBONA

Arlene Abbona would have been bald if she were a man. Baldness runs in her family, and even though she is in her early twenties, her hair was in *serious* trouble. Although a woman's hair follicle is deeper than a man's, she had severe hair loss. When I analyzed her hair, I found that she had no bulb. The root was full of oil, but her hair was dry.

Unlike many of us who eat the wrong things and drink and smoke too much, Arlene does all the right things for her body. She eats properly and exercises regularly. She thought she was using the right hair-care products, but she wasn't.

After only three weeks of my treatments, Arlene's hair came to life. It had sheen and life, and now it held a perm! That's progress. Arlene told me that she had just had a perm when she first came to me, but her hair did not look like it. Now her hair has begun to bounce with its own curl.

Before

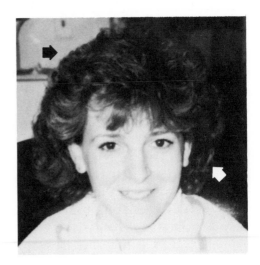

After

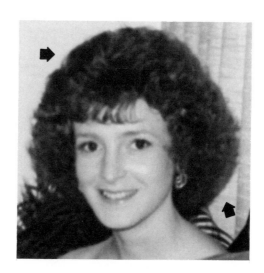

RAFAEL E. VARGAS

Rafael Vargas is in the highly competitive real-estate business in Orange County, California, and his appearance is crucial to his professional image. Consequently, his very, very oily hair and scalp, plus his rapid hair loss, posed a major problem for him. Rafael's forehead and hairline were shiny, and I was not too sure how much growth he would get. There was the beginning of serious hair-loss at his crown as well.

Before the twelve-week cycle was up, Rafael showed a major change in the texture of his hair. It was no longer slick and full of wax, and a splendid amount of peach fuzz around his hairline was clearly visible. He still has an exceptionally oily scalp, but now he knows how to keep it under control so that it doesn't suffocate his hair growth.

STEVE OBER

Steve Ober *dared* me to grow hair on his head. He had seen and heard everything about restoring hair and now he wanted full proof.

Steve was the producer of "The Morning Show" on WABC-TV in New York, where I frequently am a guest, and he had heard what I said about hair. Even seeing proof, he was dubious. When I agreed to treat his hair and scalp, he was so skeptical that he brought in his own photographer to take his pictures.

Steve had, quite frankly, very good hair, even though his scalp was waxy and his hairline was receding rapidly. He also had a circle of balding at the crown. In a matter of weeks—not even the complete twelve-week program—Steve's scalp

Before

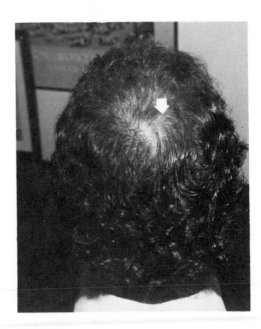

After

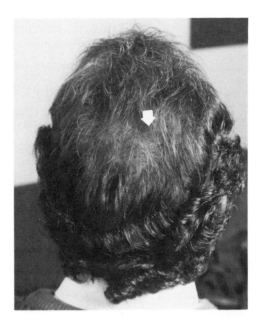

showed marked improvement, and the fuzz he had at the hairline was growing into hair. He also has regrowth through the crown.

JOHN FERRIERA

John Ferriera wouldn't let me cut his hair at first. A young model in his twenties, he is known for his Tarzan-like mane of hair. However, when John first consulted me, that mane was a bit mangled.

John's hair was thinning quickly through the top and crown. It was dry and brittle, fine and limp, even when he set it, permed it and blew it out. The hair on the back of his head suffered a lot of serious breakage. John, who likes to spend his

43

free time at the beach, also had pimples around his face and across his forehead, caused by the oils from his hair, which was always in his face.

Before

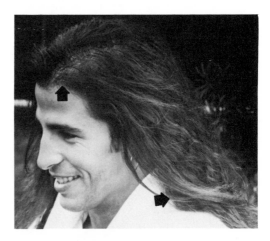

After

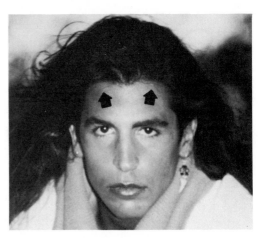

After only twelve treatments, John has almost three inches of new hair growth in back. The breakage and fallout have stopped. His hair has new growth through the crown and is much more manageable than ever before. As you can see by his pictures, the change in the texture of his hair is evident.

MITCH DOUGLAS

When Mitch Douglas began treatments, his scalp was shiny with oil and wax and his hair was lifeless. His hairline had receded until it met with the balding in his crown.

Before

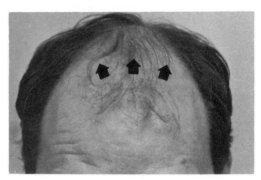

After

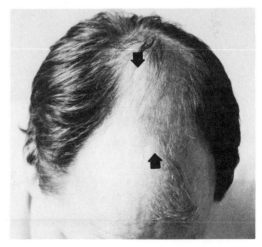

Now in his forties, Mitch who is an agent in a busy New York talent office, began to lose his hair in his late twenties. After beginning the treatments, he found that his scalp was less shiny and the waxiness began to go away, and his hair, which had been sandy brown, became darker and more full-bodied.

He now has considerable coverage through the crown, and has even begun to show new fuzz through the top, which, with continued treatments, will soon be healthy hair.

ELIOT ROSEN

When Eliot Rosen first came to me, he had absolutely no hair on top of his head. Like many men who are embarrassed by their loss of hair, he combed his up from the back to cover the balding across his crown. This trick, which calls attention to the problem rather than camouflaging it, is one of the worst things a person can do. Hair that is combed upward from the back of the head is pulled in the opposite direction from the way it naturally grows, and the sprays and lotions used to hold it in place add to the oils and wax that clog the scalp. That's the last thing a person with severe hair loss needs!

Before

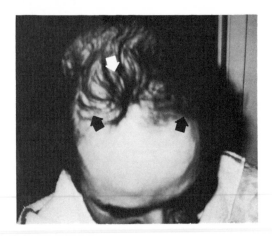

After

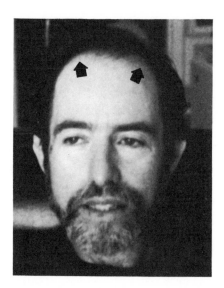

Eliot's hair was limp and dry and his scalp was quite waxy with oily buildup from his sebaceous glands. I cut his hair close to the scalp, relieving the tension caused by forcing his hair to go against nature, and then taught him how to clean his scalp and hair, as well as how to stimulate the blood flow to his roots.

He quickly began to show new growth, which pleased him greatly. Eliot was so excited about his new hair and its continued regrowth that he went on television with me several times to demonstrate these treatments.

RON RONAN

A massage therapist with a busy Manhattan practice as well as one in suburban Connecticut, Ron had begun to lose his hair at a rapid pace, both at the crown and through his hairline. Ron was not happy about the condition of his hair, either, which was very dry. Within a week of beginning treatments, Ron showed marked improvement in the condition of his hair. It had more body and sheen, and its texture was visibly different, with softer wave and curl. Within a month, Ron had noticeable growth at the hairline as well as through the crown.

Before

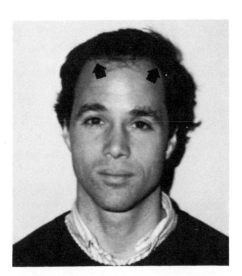

After

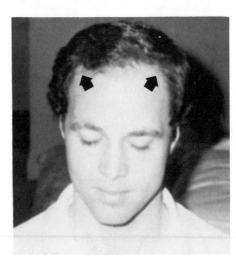

DR. BENJAMIN COLIMORE

April 3, 1987

Dear Riquette,

I want to tell you how pleased and gratified I am with the treatments you have given me on my skin and the products which you have prepared for my skin and hair. The change has been remarkable and so immediate that I could scarcely believe my eyes.

Thank you for your expertise, and for the sensational research that went into your products, all based on natural foods and herbs. What a wonderful service you are rendering to both men and women who want better skin and hair without the irritations of chemicals.

Thank you so much! And keep up the good work!

Gratefully yours,

Benjamin Colimore, Ph.D.

Dr. Benjamin Colimore is a respected nutritionist and author who formerly practiced in Los Angeles. Now living in Colorado, he continues to use my program to keep his hair healthy and to halt hair loss. Dr. Colimore is an advocate of my skincare program as well.

REBECCA FOLSOM

By the time she found her way to my clinic, Rebecca Folsom had tried everything on the market to "fix" her thin, fine hair. Because of an underactive thyroid condition that plagued her for nine years, her hair grew very slowly. It was so fragile when I began treating it that it would break at a touch.

At first, Rebecca would not let me cut her hair, much less perm or color it, for fear it would be damaged even further. She had been treated for a *dry* scalp condition, which was quite wrong. Her scalp was really very oily, and the products she was using were making matters worse.

Before

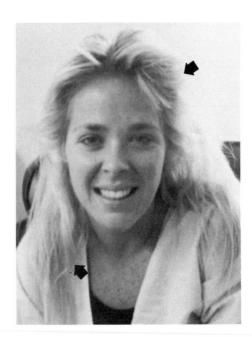

After

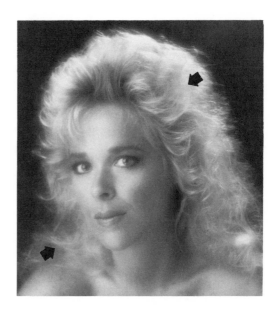

Rebecca is so pleased with the results of my treatments that in less than twelve weeks she has allowed me to brighten the color of her dishwater blond hair and trim some of the brittle, damaged ends. "I certainly wouldn't be coming back if it didn't work," she explains. Before coming to see me, Rebecca had tried everything, going from doctor to doctor, from tricologist to tricologist all over the world. "I went to almost every hair specialist I ever heard of, and my hair only got worse... until now."

4
TAKE A GOOD LOOK FOR YOURSELF
Watch Your Peach Fuzz Turn into Hair

||||||||||||||||||||||||||||||||||||||||||||||||||||||||||||||||||||||||||||||

Your memory may be able to fool you, but photos won't, which is why you must begin to keep a record of your progress. As trivial as it may appear, it is almost as vital to the success of the program as is your commitment to your treatments.

Right now you are probably thinking that you will be able to remember how you look today, but I promise you that you won't. Your memory is *not* a reliable record; in fact, it will trick you.

You see yourself in the mirror every day, so you are accustomed to your hair. Without photographs taken at regular intervals to record any changes in your hair's growth and texture, as well as its color, you truly won't be able to see your progress.

Set up your own confidential photographic record to jar your memory and to bolster your confidence when you become impatient. Remember, you did not lose your hair overnight—even if it seems that way. For most people, hair loss is a gradual process occurring over a period of months, if not years. You cannot expect it to grow back overnight!

These may be some of the most important pictures you have ever taken, so I want you to do exactly what I say.

First, find a picture of yourself *before* your hair loss began. If you haven't kept a box of snapshots on the top shelf of your hall closet, you can use the picture from your high school yearbook or from an old driver's license or passport. Better yet, ask your mother. I'm sure *she* has a photograph you can use.

You will *never* look that way again, but it's an excellent reminder of what you are shooting for! How much hair will grow back depends upon the condition of your scalp and the amount and condition of the fuzz you have.

New photographs should be taken from a vantage point that best exposes your bald spots and receding hairline. This is no time for vanity! It is essential that you show your baldness in order to be able to recognize the changes that will take place.

Ask a friend to take pictures that focus on your progress. Better yet, get a friend or loved one to join you in the program. You can each give the treatments to the other and take the pictures showing the other's progress.

If you comb your hair across the top of your head to cover your bare spots, take two photos: one that shows the way you style your hair every day, and another with the long, covering hair held out of the way to expose the full extent of your hair loss.

David, now in his thirties, started losing his hair in his early twenties. He was pulling a section of hair up and over from the back to cover the baldness at the crown and across the top of his head. Take a photo that shows how you usually style your hair.

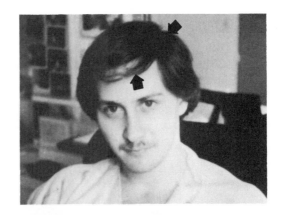

When David combed his hair back from his forehead, his *open* hairline was clearly visible. David's hair and scalp were oily, and his roots thin and weak. You too must take a picture that shows the *total* extent of your baldness. David lived through it . . . and so can you!

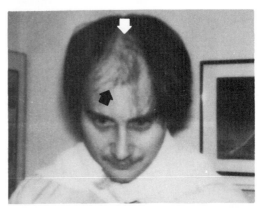

In addition to the wedge of balding from the hairline in front, David also had a circle of loss at the crown. In this picture you can see the irregular length on the right. This hair was combed up, across the crown, as part of his camouflage. Notice how the oiliness is reflected in the hair texture.

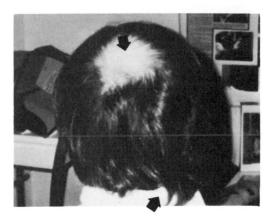

55

David's hair growth was dramatic. In this "after" picture, you can see clearly how new hair is growing through the crown as well as across the hairline. Remember, these pictures were taken with my little instant camera so that we could have a record of David's progress for his eyes only. Hardly studio-quality photography, they still show the improvement in his hair and scalp.

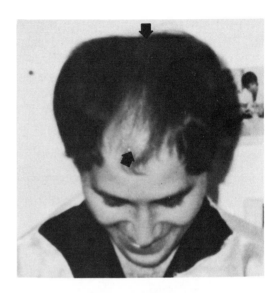

See how the crown was almost completely covered after David had done the treatments for twelve weeks. He continued with the program and has continued to show progress. His hair texture has completely changed. It is darker, fuller, and incredibly healthier than ever before. Don't you want to see how much regrowth you will have in only twelve weeks?

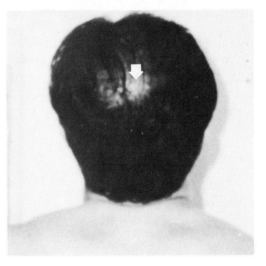

If your hairline is receding, pictures should be taken from the front, looking down. If you have a circle of balding at the crown associated with male pattern baldness, have pictures taken from the back, slightly above the head.

A word of warning: Don't hold the camera too close to your head. The light from your flash will "burn" out any detail in the photographs and you won't be able to see the hair and fuzz in them. Shoot from three feet away for best results.

Whenever possible, take your pictures from the same position, with the same exposure settings and lighting.

Because hair grows at different rates for different people, I am asking you to take pictures before you begin treatments and then every three weeks during the initial twelve-week program.

If you do not see immediate, rapid results, do not be discouraged and give up. As I have warned you, you didn't lose your hair overnight. Stay on the program, *doing every step exactly as I instruct you to do it*, following the entire treatment schedule for your hair, scalp and skin for twelve weeks.

I promise you that within three weeks you will begin to see results. Ordinarily, hair grows approximately one half inch per month. With these treatments, the growth rate will be considerably faster.

However, the treatments will not work if you leave them in the bottles or on the shelf. You have to put them on your head to get results.

You have nothing to lose and everything to gain. Don't you deserve it?

5
HOW TO GROW HAIR IN 12 WEEKS
Riquette's Hair Rejuvenation Program

||||||||||||||||||||||||||||||||||||||||||||||||||||||||||||||||||||||||||

Let me repeat my promise to you:

If you have any peach fuzz on your scalp, I *guarantee* three things: first, I will turn that peach fuzz into hair in twelve weeks; second, I will totally transform the texture of your hair; and third, I will stop further hair loss.

You have heard my promise and seen the pictures of some of my clients. If you still question the success of the program, let me introduce you to John Edwards.

At his class reunion, John was voted the man who had lost

John Edwards pulled this snapshot from his family scrapbook to show how much hair he had lost and how shiny his scalp was before he began treatments. I tried to persuade him not to waste his money on the program. I was unwilling to promise him any results at all.

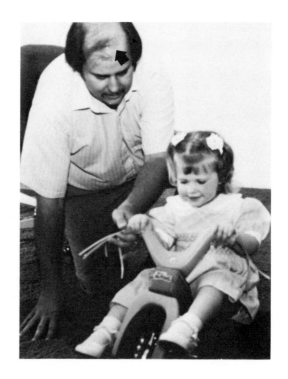

the most hair. When he started coming to my clinic, he had only a few wisps of hair at the top of his head. I could neither see nor feel any appreciable peach fuzz on his scalp. It was so shiny with waxy buildup that I refused to guarantee *any* results. In fact, I tried to discourage him from beginning treatments at all.

John would have none of it. He had heard so much about me and how well my program worked that he was willing to gamble twelve weeks of his time and money for *any* improvement. He said that he would be willing to stop his chronic hair loss and nothing more!

A salesman in a high-pressure job, John had gained weight and lost considerable hair over the past few years. He didn't feel that his baldness was holding him back in his job, but he did believe he would feel better if he had more hair.

At the time of John's first consultation with me, his hair was so oily that it hung in strings against the back of his head. I could barely detect any fuzz at all on his crown.

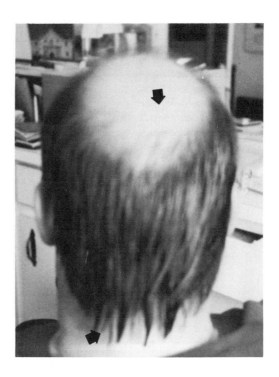

I agreed to begin treatments with John's understanding that I could not promise results.

Within six weeks we saw noticeable improvements in John's hair. His drop-out rate fell drastically, and the oiliness in both his scalp and hair subsided. His forehead and scalp were no longer waxy and his hair was no longer greasy.

By the end of the initial twelve weeks, new hair—follicles that had been "sleeping" beneath his wax-clogged scalp—began to grow. Now John is looking forward to his next reunion and the very real possibility that he will no longer be the class baldy!

How much regrowth you will have, I cannot predict. Results vary from person to person, sometimes without apparent reason. I have been surprised by clients like John, who, at first examination, appear destined to fail but have experienced al-

It did take more than twelve weeks to grow hair on John's head, but within six months he had amazing regrowth. The texture of his hair had completely changed, and his scalp, rather than being coated with oil and wax, was smooth and supple.

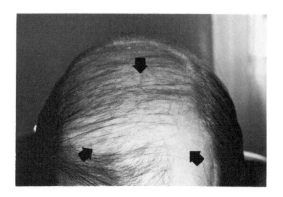

most complete coverage. Others, however, who seem far more promising, sometimes do little more than stop further drastic loss and improve the quality of their existing hair.

I will not promise anyone *total* regrowth, but I will assure the best possible results with the hair you have left. You must have peach fuzz to grow hair.

By now you have studied the condition of your root and hair and have taken stock of your general health and lifestyle —all the factors that figure into the condition of your hair and scalp.

Now it is time to look at your commitment to this program. I can't force you to do it—that's up to you—but I can explain what you will be doing.

The program I have created takes twelve weeks to complete. During this time, you will use seven special treatments for your scalp and hair. Some are to be done daily, others once a week.

Recipes for these treatments are simple to follow. Made from ingredients that are easily purchased in grocery stores, pharmacies and health food shops, they are also inexpensive to use, costing at least half as much as other programs and drug therapies per month, and producing far more satisfactory, *long-term* results.

When people protest that they can't cook, I tell them that all

As John's hair begins to grow, new fuzz has begun to push through. Now he has hope for even more coverage.

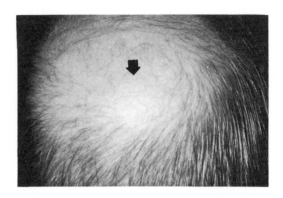

they need to know is how to boil water. That's about as complicated as these recipes get.

The time involvement per day is minimal, especially once you get into the routine. You will massage stimulating oils—the Basic Stimulator—into your scalp every night at bedtime. In the morning you will wash your hair, using a Scalp Shampoo and a Hair Shampoo, and follow each washing with a simple Protective Sealing Lotion to detangle your hair and restore the acid balance to your hair and scalp. A Volume Enhancer is used to replace commercially prepared styling products.

This special treatment takes no more time than washing your hair with commercially prepared products, and shows incredible results.

Once a week you will use the Super Stimulator to increase circulation to the root of your hair and follow this with my famous Slougher Cocktail, which dissolves wax and dead cells that have adhered to the scalp, and a third scalp treatment, the Mud Pack, which absorbs excess oils.

After rinsing these scalp treatments away, you will apply a special Protein Pack that bonds with your hair shaft to repair and protect the hair itself, then complete the treatment by washing with both scalp and hair cleansers and using the Protective Sealing Lotion and Volume Enhancer.

THE COMPLETE PROGRAM OF HAIR AND SKIN CARE TREATMENTS

Hair Program

EVERY MORNING
  Brush Hair
  Scalp Shampoo
    (page 88)
  Hair Shampoo
    (pages 88–89)
  Rinse with tepid water
  Protective Sealing
    Lotion (page 92)
  Volume Enhancer
    (pages 96–97)
  Wash hairbrush and
    combs

EVERY EVENING
  Basic Stimulator
    (page 72)

ONCE A WEEK
  Super Stimulator
    (page 73)
  Slougher Cocktail
    (page 77)
  Mud Pack (pages 80–81)
  Protein Pack (page 84)
  Scalp Shampoo
  Hair Shampoo
  Protective Sealing Lotion
  Volume Enhancer

Skin Program

EVERY MORNING
  Deep Pore
    Morning Cleanser
    (page 114)
  Toner (page 115)
  Moisturizer (page 115)

EVERY EVENING
  Nightly Cleanser
    (page 114)
  Toner
  Moisturizer

ONCE A WEEK
  Mud Mask (page 116)
  Rinse
  Toner
  Moisturizer

Each treatment is explained in detail in the chapters that follow, and I have prepared a chart for your reference that tells you what to do and when. Most of my clients post their charts in their bathrooms to record their progress.

These scalp and hair treatments are augmented by a simple skin-care program to create a balance between your scalp and your face—especially your forehead. These treatments are listed on the chart, too.

My only request is that, should you choose to follow my Hair Rejuvenation Program, you follow every step and every recipe *exactly as written* for the next twelve weeks. Make no substitutions or omissions.

Some of my clients team up with a friend, or several friends, and create a support group, having weekly hair parties to do the program together. Others make hair care a family affair, enrolling everyone—including the children—in the program. Remember, you are *never* too young to take care of your hair, scalp and skin!

The treatments, I must add, are habit-forming. After a week, you will get into the swing of things. "Doing things" to your hair and scalp, as well as your skin, will become second nature within a couple of weeks. It is as easy to take care of yourself as not to do so.

The herbs that I have chosen for the basic program are simple, pure products known through the ages to have special properties that encourage hair growth and healthy skin. They are very powerful, especially when used as I have requested.

After you have followed the program for twelve weeks without varying the recipes as written, I invite the adventurers among you to join me in exploring other herbal treasures known to benefit the body. The final chapter of this book is full of treatments to supplement the original series so that you can experience more benefits of natural hair and skin care.

You have probably heard of everything on the basic shopping list. Much of what I ask you to buy will come from your corner pharmacy or neighborhood grocery store. Other ingredients—the essential oils and dried herbs, roots, seeds, flowers and organics—can be found in health food stores and herb shops. Check the Yellow Pages of your telephone directory if you don't know where to look. Try under Botanicals, Health Food Stores, Herbs, Nature/Natural Ingredients, Oils/ Essential, Pharmacies/Natural or Homeopathic.

If you are still unable to find what you need nearby, there are some outstanding distributors who fulfill mail or telephone orders. Check the Source Guide on page 159 for a list of suppliers who will be able to provide the necessary ingredients.

BUYING AND STORING HERBS

Fresh herbs may be wonderful for cooking, but for our purposes their potency is too difficult to measure. For example, you would need 4 ounces of parsley leaves, if not more, to produce the same concentration as in 1 ounce of dried parsley. For a bark or a root, which has a much lower water content than a leafy plant, the ratio might be only 1¼ ounces of the fresh product to 1 ounce of the dried.

It takes a lot of training and many, many years of practice to become proficient in measuring fresh herbs and plants for cosmetic use, so, to keep things simple, all the ingredients used in these recipes will be dried, rather than fresh or powdered.

While measurements are not critical to the preparation of herbal cosmetics, I want you to stick to the recipes exactly as I have written them so that you will experience the results I have promised. See page 157 for a table of weights and measurements that will help you when preparing your treatments.

I suggest that you buy herbs and plants in the smallest possible amounts, unless I indicate otherwise on the basic shopping list. You can always purchase more as you need them.

Keep your ingredients in small *glass* jars with tight-fitting lids. Save empty spice jars so you won't have to buy new ones. Label each container as you fill it, then store it in a cool, dry place—never over the stove, or the herbs will become too dry. Measure them with dry, nonmetallic instruments if possible. I will tell you how to store and label the individual treatments with each recipe so there will be no confusion.

Here is *everything* you will need to purchase for the complete hair and skin care program detailed in the chapters that follow.

BASIC SHOPPING LIST

Basics
  Alka-Seltzer (36-tablet box)
  Alum (small container)
  Aspirin (large bottle; generic is fine)
  Castile soap*
  Castor oil (odorless)
  Cayenne pepper (3½-ounce container)
  Distilled water
  Egg (one per week)
  Glycerine and rosewater (4-ounce bottle)
  Honey
  Powdered milk
  Protein nutritional supplement powder (any brand; unflavored if possible)
  Sesame oil (1 pint, any quality brand)
  Vinegar (large bottle; apple cider or, if hair is white or light blond, white vinegar)
  Vodka (any inexpensive brand)
  White iodine

---

*If possible, buy liquid castile soap without additives or, if not available, a cake of pure castile soap and dissolve shavings in 1 quart of hot water. If neither is available, Dr. Bronner's Pure Castile Soap with Almond Oil is an excellent alternative. Next best is Dr. Bronner's Pure Castile Soap with Peppermint Oil.

Essential Oils
Almond (1 ounce; substitute sesame oil if almond oil is not available)
Basil (if available)*
Lavender (2 ounces)
Lemon (2 ounces)
Rosemary (3 ounces)
Wheat germ (1 ounce)

Dried Herbs, Roots, Seeds and Organics†
Basil leaves
Chamomile flowers
Flaxseeds (4 ounces)
Fuller's earth (12 ounces)
Lavender
Nettles
Neutral henna (12 ounces)
Rosemary leaves
Sage
Thyme

Equipment
Amber bottles (2- or 3-ounce size), preferably with glass dropper top. Do not recycle a nose drops bottle unless you can *thoroughly* sterilize both bottle and dropper. You can purchase a new bottle and dropper from your pharmacist for a dollar or less.
Blender (optional)

---

*Natural basil oil is often difficult to find and is frequently quite expensive. It is the best stimulator known, but rosemary oil is a viable substitute. Buy 2-ounce minimum if available.

†I recommend buying dried herbs and plants by the scoop, unless I have specified a definite amount or this is less than the minimum order allowed. Buy powdered herbs *only* if whole dried leaves or flowers are not available.

Bottles and jars (glass, preferably amber), assorted sizes, with tight-fitting lids or corks.

Bowls (glass or enamel), assorted sizes

Cheesecloth (for straining and for wrapping hairbrush)

Eye dropper (glass), if not included with amber bottle

Magnifying glass

Measuring cup (glass)

Mortar and pestle (optional, can be improvised)

Pastry brush

Pots with lids (enamel, assorted sizes)

Soft toothbrush (the softer the better)

Strainer (fine mesh)

Teakettle

Waterproof labels

Wooden spoons

PUTTING YOUR HERBS TO USE

Once you have purchased all your supplies, you must learn how to use them. As I tell my clients, all you need to know is how to boil water.

The recipes for each treatment will tell you which herbs you will use and the amounts required for each. The way you use these herbs is the same for each recipe: you make an *infusion*, which is merely a strong tea, made by pouring 2 cups of boiling water into a prewarmed pot and adding an ounce or more of the dried herbs. Cover and allow the infusion to steep for at least 10 minutes—longer if you can—to extract all of the wonderful properties of the herbs. Strain and cool before using for treatments.

Later, when you become more adventurous and have completed the basic twelve-week program, you can expand your hair-care treatments with more complicated recipes that may call for you to use roots, barks and hard seeds. To extract the goodness from these tougher parts of the plants, you must make a *decoction*. Put an ounce or more of the plant parts into an enamel pot and cover with 2 cups of water. Cover the pot and bring to a boil. Reduce the heat and simmer for at least 20 minutes. Steep 30 minutes and strain the liquid into a jar.

When using herbs, you may want to crush the leaves between your palms before tossing them into the water, or mash your barks, roots, chips and seeds with a mortar and pestle to soften them just a bit before making a decoction.

After you have made your treatments, discard any leftover infusions and decoctions. Your purpose is fresh, natural products.

ON YOUR MARK, GET SET, LET'S GO!

Read the program through, from start to finish. Then go back and read it again.

Now you can prepare your treatments! Follow each recipe step by step, and label each container as you fill it to prevent confusion later on.

Store lotions and potions in glass containers with tight-fitting lids. Ideally, you should use amber glass jars and bottles, but clear glass is acceptable. Keep your products in a cool, dry, dark place. Light and heat will break down herbs and natural products. Some herbal cosmetic purists insist upon using amber containers and then covering the bottles with paper!

My system for retarding spoilage is even simpler: prepare quantities that can be used up in a short amount of time. Dried herbs and pure oils have a longer shelf life than herbal compounds.

Here's everything you will need to know about how to make and use the treatments I have created to start on the road to healthy hair, scalp and skin.

6
REACHING THE ROOT

Treatment 1:
The Stimulators

||||||||||||||||||||||||||||||||||||||||||||||||||||||||||||||||||||||||||||

If healthy, strong hair is to grow, the scalp must be completely free of excess oils and dead cells, and the roots must be well fed. This means that blood must flow freely through the scalp. To accomplish this, I want you to massage special oils which I have chosen because they are well known for their abilities to stimulate blood circulation as well as hair growth. Do this *every single night* at bedtime, without fail.

As you massage these fragrant, stimulating oils into your scalp, you will feel a tingling sensation. This is caused by the blood which is now circulating through your scalp like never before. It is important that you massage your forehead and neck as well as your scalp. Make sure that the oils actually penetrate your skin. They have important work to do!

The program I have created for you includes a Basic Stimulator, which is used nightly, and a Super Stimulator, applied once a week.

BASIC STIMULATOR

Apply every night

6 teaspoons rosemary oil
3 teaspoons basil oil (if available; other-
wise use 2 teaspoons rosemary oil)
3 teaspoons lavender oil
2 teaspoons lemon oil

Put the oils into an amber bottle with a glass dropper top. Close tightly and shake well to mix. Label.

Pour two teaspoons of Basic Stimulator into a glass bowl. Massage into your scalp with your fingertips. Divide your hair into small sections at the hairline and work from the forehead to the crown. Concentrate on the areas of balding, then distribute the remainder over the rest of your head, hairline and ends of hair.

Leave the Basic Stimulator on your head overnight. Most of the oils will have been absorbed by your hair and scalp, so you need not be concerned about getting oil on your pillow. If you still want to play it safe, cover your pillow with a terry cloth towel.

In the morning, wash out with the Hair and Scalp Shampoos, following the recipes on pages 88–89.

As I explained, the Basic Stimulator is a *nightly* treatment and the Super Stimulator is a *weekly* treatment. *Do them both.*

The Super Stimulator is exactly what the name implies: a

powerful scalp stimulator. It is to be used once a week in conjunction with the three other special treatments: the Slougher Cocktail, the Mud Pack and the Protein Pack.

This once-a-week stimulation treatment is not a replacement for the nightly applications of the Basic Stimulator.

SUPER STIMULATOR

Apply once a week

2 teaspoons Basic Stimulator
2 teaspoons basil oil (if available; otherwise use 2 teaspoons rosemary oil)
1 teaspoon white iodine
½ teaspoon castor oil

Put ingredients in an amber glass bottle with a glass dropper top. Close tightly and shake to mix thoroughly. Label.

Apply Super Stimulator to the scalp in the same way as the Basic Stimulator. Massage for 10 minutes, then leave on the head 10 minutes longer.

Do not rinse.

Continue with Treatment 2 of the Weekly Program—The Slougher Cocktail.

7

TO YOUR HEALTH!
Treatment 2:
The Slougher Cocktail

||||||||||||||||||||||||||||||||||||||||||||||||||||||||||||||||||||||||||

I introduced my Slougher Cocktail to the public on national television—on "The Merv Griffin Show," to be exact—when I applied it to the famous bald head of Don Rickles. I have demonstrated it on "Late Night with David Letterman" as well as other shows, and no matter how many times I have shown it on TV or talked about it in interviews, public response has been overwhelming. People love it!

Sloughing is the most effective way to dissolve wax buildup and remove dead cells caused by improper washing and in-

Apply my fabulous Slougher Cocktail with a soft toothbrush. Dip your brush into the bowl and, starting at the hairline, work your way back to the crown. Once your entire scalp is covered, massage Slougher into the ends of your hair to dissolve shampoo residue.

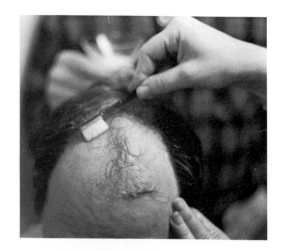

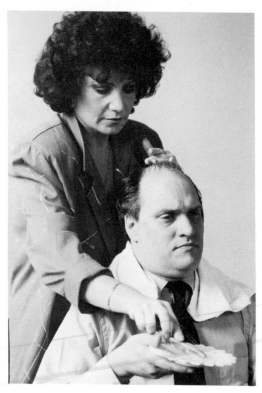

sufficient rinsing, as well as not brushing properly. These impurities, as well as dust and pollution, clog the pores of the scalp and smother the root before the hair has a chance to grow.

Applied to the scalp with a soft toothbrush, the Slougher Cocktail loosens scaling such as dandruff and seborrhea while stimulating blood circulation through the scalp.

Be sure to use every ingredient in the Slougher Cocktail recipe because each one has a specific purpose, and together they work to cleanse your scalp totally.

SLOUGHER COCKTAIL

Apply once a week

¼ cup vodka
10 aspirin tablets
2 Alka-Seltzer tablets
2 teaspoons Scalp Shampoo (page 88)
1 teaspoon cayenne pepper

In a small glass bowl, gently stir all the ingredients together until the tablets are dissolved.

Section your hair from the hairline, a little at a time. Using a soft toothbrush, apply the Slougher to your scalp and rub in a gentle, circular motion until your entire head is covered with Slougher. *Do not scrub too hard; you are not scouring a pot.*

Once you have covered your scalp, massage the remaining Slougher into the ends of your hair. This will dissolve any oily residue there.

Apply next treatment without rinsing this one.

8

A REAL DIAMOND IN THE ROUGH

Treatment 3:
The Mud Pack

||||||||||||||||||||||||||||||||||||||||||||||||||||||||||||||||||||||||||||||

Beauty-conscious women have known about the value of mud and clay in caring for the skin and hair since the days of Cleopatra, at least. Now I am going to share this secret with all of you!

When I speak of mud, I am not talking about the mud that children track in from the backyard, but a mixture of fuller's earth and neutral henna.

Fuller's earth is a highly absorbent substance made of very

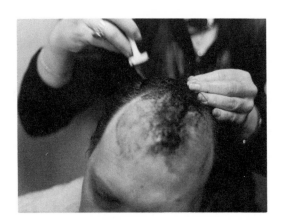

The Mud Pack draws excess oils from your scalp and keeps the sebaceous glands from overproducing. Apply the pack, which should be the consistency of oatmeal, with a pastry brush.

pure clay and a natural, sandlike powder. Its gentle, absorbent quality is the very reason I use it.

The other ingredient in this very special recipe is neutral henna. This famous Egyptian herbal compound has been used in cosmetics and medicines for thousands and thousands of years. It makes an excellent hair wash, rinse or dye, depending upon the strength of the solution you use. The powdered leaves can be mixed with other herbs to make different-colored natural semipermanent dyes.

For our purposes, we will be using neutral (color-free) henna. It leaves no color in the hair shaft but does *wonderful* things to the body of your hair.

Both fuller's earth and neutral henna absorb the oils from the scalp and act as healing agents for an irritated scalp.

MUD PACK

Apply once a week

1 cup fuller's earth
1 cup neutral henna

Combine fuller's earth and neutral henna in a plastic bag with a zipper top or in a glass jar with a tight-fitting lid. Shake powders together to mix thoroughly and use as necessary.

In a glass bowl, combine 2 tablespoons Mud Pack powder with 2 to 3 tablespoons boiling water. Add enough water to make a smooth, thick paste the consistency of oatmeal.

Using a pastry brush, apply the Mud Pack to your head. Work into your scalp and then rub into the ends of your hair. Do not worry about massaging the mud into your scalp because it is too thick. Leave on for 30 minutes.

Rinse thoroughly with warm or cool water.

9

HIGH PROTEIN
HEALTH SHAKE

Treatment 4:
The Protein Pack

|||||||||||||||||||||||||||||||||||||||||||||||||||||||||||||||||||||||||||||

If you use a protein pack, you will never need a so-called cream rinse again! Such rinses are used to detangle hair after washing, especially if the hair has been abused and damaged and has a rough cuticle or exterior. Rather than correcting this damage, these rinses or conditioning products act as filler, coating the rough edges and ridges in the hair shaft. The emollients in these products are waxy and oily, so it's no wonder that, by lunchtime, your hair looks and feels like it hasn't been washed!

My Protein Pack, however, will bond the scales of the cuticle to the shaft, creating a smooth and tangle-free head of hair. As I have explained, hair is 97 percent protein, and very difficult to alter. In fact, nothing in the world—except another protein —can actually fuse with the medulla to repair any damage.

In addition to this first-aid function, the Protein Pack bonds with the shaft to strengthen it and add resilience.

Apply the Protein Pack once a week—right after the Mud Pack—using a pastry brush. If your hair is especially dry or damaged, use the Protein Pack twice a week. Be sure to work it into the ends of your hair.

PROTEIN PACK

Apply once a week,
twice a week
for dry or damaged hair

2 tablespoons protein nutritional supplement powder
1 egg yolk
1 tablespoon cold-pressed sesame oil
2 to 3 tablespoons hot water

In a glass or enamel bowl, stir the ingredients together. Use enough hot water to dissolve the powder and thoroughly blend egg and oil. It should be the consistency of a loose paste.

Using a pastry brush, apply it to your hair, paying attention to the ends, then work it into the hairline.

Wrap your hair in a plastic bag or cover it with a plastic shower cap and then a warm, moist towel to keep your head warm. Leave on for 10 minutes before rinsing with warm water.

10

YOU'LL NEVER *JUST* WASH YOUR HAIR AGAIN

Treatment 5: Scalp Shampoo and Hair Shampoo

||||||||||||||||||||||||||||||||||||||||||||||||||||||||||||||||||||||||

Until now, probably no one has ever told you to wash your hair every day with two *different* shampoos.

Well, I am telling you to do so.

One is for your scalp, and the other is for your hair.

This is because your hair and your scalp are entirely different, with entirely different requirements from a cleansing product. Each cleanser has a specific purpose. Used in conjunction, they clean both hair and scalp to perfection.

The Scalp Shampoo supports the Slougher in keeping the

scalp clean. Daily cleansing with this shampoo, along with the weekly Slougher treatments, will eliminate any impurities that stick to the scalp, such as dust and dirt, as well as oil, which, if left on the scalp, will clog the pores. It also has an astringent, antiseptic effect on the scalp, balancing and bringing it to a normal state.

The Hair Shampoo removes impurities and dirt from the hair shaft itself, gently cleansing and adding body to the hair without any drying effect.

Too many all-purpose shampoos available today are so busy trying to do everything with one application that the primary purpose of a shampoo—to wash and cleanse the hair and scalp—gets lost in the shuffle. How can one product clean an oily scalp and condition dry hair at the same time?

THE RIQUETTE WAY TO SHAMPOO

My clients tease me and say there is a wrong way and a Riquette way of doing things. Well, since my way of doing these treatments *works*, they might be right!

With this in mind, I am going to teach you the Riquette way to wash your hair.

You will, of course, apply the Basic Stimulator (page 72) to your scalp every night, massage it in until the oils have been absorbed, get a good night's sleep and awaken relaxed and energetic in the morning to a magnificent shower and shampoo. Since you already do this—shower and shampoo, that is—you won't be disrupting your morning routine in the least by using two different shampoos.

Use the Scalp Shampoo first, rinse with tepid water, then use the Hair Shampoo, rinse again with tepid water, finish with the Protective Sealing Lotion and, if you need a styling aid, use the Volume Enhancer, described in the next two chapters.

This shampooing technique should be used daily.

If you work out or swim during the day and wash your hair a second time, use only the Hair Shampoo for the second washing.

MAKING YOUR SHAMPOOS

The key ingredient in these shampoos is castile soap, in liquid or lotion form. Castile is a fine, hard, unscented soap, usually white or cream-colored, named for the region of Spain where it was first made.

If you are unable to find liquid or lotion castile soap, you can easily make your own by shaving a bar of pure castile soap, preferably made with olive oil and no additives, into a quart of hot water. Let it simmer over low heat until all the soap chips have dissolved, or cover and let it sit overnight until they have dissolved. This viscous lotion is the basis for both the Scalp Shampoo and the Hair Shampoo.

If you are unable to purchase pure castile soap in any of its commercially prepared forms—liquid, powder or bar—you can use Dr. Bronner's Pure Castile Soap with Almond Oil. See my explanation of these alternatives in the Basic Shopping List (page 67).

You will prepare the herbs used in each of these shampoos by making an infusion or tea for each, and straining the liquid into ½ cup of liquid castile soap. (For a refresher course in making infusions, see page 69.)

SCALP SHAMPOO

Apply once a day

1 heaping tablespoon crushed basil leaves
1 heaping tablespoon lavender flowers
1 heaping tablespoon rosemary leaves
3 cups boiling water
½ cup liquid castile soap

Make an infusion of the herbs and boiling water. Cover and let steep for a minimum of 10 minutes.

Strain the infusion into ½ cup liquid castile soap.

Store in a nonbreakable bottle. Label.

Use 1 teaspoon Scalp Shampoo per washing. Apply to wet hair. Massage into scalp, adding a little water at a time to work into a lather.

Rinse thoroughly, using tepid water. Then wash with Hair Shampoo.

HAIR SHAMPOO

Apply once a day

1 heaping tablespoon nettles
1 heaping tablespoon crushed sage
1 heaping tablespoon chamomile flowers
3 cups boiling water
½ cup liquid castile soap

Make an infusion of the herbs and boiling water. Cover and let steep for a minimum of 10 minutes.

Strain the infusion into ½ cup liquid castile soap.

Store in a nonbreakable bottle. Label.

Use only 1 teaspoon of this highly concentrated shampoo per washing, massaging it gently into your hair. Rinse thoroughly with tepid water until water runs clear.

As a final rinse, use my Protective Sealing Lotion, described in the next chapter, to restore the acid mantle of the hair and scalp.

After using these very special shampoo products, you will not be pleased with most of the products sold in stores. I've had clients tell me that their old brands of shampoo make their hair feel gummy and sticky after they have been using my highly concentrated scalp and hair cleansers. They leave no residue on your hair, so you won't need to be changing shampoos every few months.

Make enough of your private-label scalp and hair shampoos to have for your gym bag so you can use them after working out, and for your travel bag so you will have them with you while you're on the road.

11

GIVE YOUR HAIR A GRAND FINALE!

Treatment 6:
The Protective Sealing Lotion

||||||||||||||||||||||||||||||||||||||||||||||||||||||||||||||||||||||

The grand finale to my daily treatment regimen is a Protective Sealing Lotion that will flatten the hair's cuticle and restore the 2 percent acid mantle to the hair and scalp.

This is a delicate balance that is easily disturbed, especially if there is any soapy residue left in the hair and on the scalp after washing. The result of this simple treatment will be hair that is squeaky clean and absolutely shimmering with life. Clients often tell me how different their hair *feels*, and especially that it doesn't have that slick, coated feeling it has after washing with most commercially packaged shampoos and rinsing agents.

Wash your hair according to my instructions, and rinse it until the water runs clear after your second lathering with the Hair Shampoo. As a final rinse, poor a diluted solution of Protective Sealing Lotion and warm water through your hair.

Once again, you are working with a highly concentrated product, so a little goes a l-o-n-g way. The following recipe makes enough to last for more than two weeks.

PROTECTIVE SEALING LOTION

Apply once a day

32-ounce bottle apple cider vinegar
1 heaping tablespoon rosemary
1 heaping tablespoon sage
1 heaping tablespoon nettles
1 heaping tablespoon basil
1 heaping tablespoon chamomile

Crush herbs gently with a mortar and pestle, or rub them between the palms of your hands to break them up a little.

Heat the apple cider vinegar in an enamel or glass pot. Add the herbs. Cover and simmer over low heat for 30 minutes.

Cool, then strain and funnel the liquid back into the vinegar bottle for safekeeping. Label and store in the refrigerator.

Don't forget to label your Protective Sealing Lotion. Nothing in it would harm you, but I don't think this souped-up vinegar would be very tasty in a salad dressing.

Mix ¼ cup Protective Sealing Lotion with 1 quart tepid water. Pour through your hair as a final rinse.

If you are afraid the vinegar smell might be too strong, you can use a little clear water before toweling dry. My experience has been that all vinegar smell disappears once your hair is dry.

Briskly rub your hair and scalp with terry cloth towels or, better yet, "mittens" made of terry cloth. This will not only absorb much of the excess water but will also stimulate circulation in your scalp.

Comb your hair with your fresh, clean comb and then style. To increase your hair's body and provide added protection to new growth when drying either hair or scalp, use my Volume Enhancer.

12

AND NOW FOR A STANDING OVATION!

Treatment 7: The Volume Enhancer

||||||||||||||||||||||||||||||||||||||||||||||||||||||||||||||||||||||||

Styling aids—from mousses to gels and from blow dryers to styling wands—are as common as ice cream and cake nowadays. Everyone uses them! We have our hair *styled* rather than just cut or barbered. We apply colors and rinses, perms and straighteners—anything that we feel might make us more attractive.

Anyone who has hair and scalp problems, especially severe hair loss from either male pattern baldness or alopecia areata, will try just about anything on earth to make his or her hair look better or thicker or restore lost hair while maintaining what hair is left.

Ironically, the latest additions to this growing trend in hair care and styling, especially mousses and gels, can be brutally damaging. In fact, they can be almost as harmful to both hair and scalp as that "greasy kid stuff" and oily tonic of the fifties and sixties or the alcohol-filled grooming aids that Grandpa might have used. Most of the popularly marketed products have alcohol in them. Others, though they are "alcohol-free," are full of chemicals that take their toll on the delicate composition of the hair.

Hair-styling lotions make the hair more pliable and keep it in place. This is accomplished by coating the hair shaft and soaking the layers of the cuticle. Strong chemicals, such as alcohol, can literally damage the interior structure of the hair if they are misused.

Once again, I turned to nature for a styling aid that cannot over-dry or harm your hair, despite the fact that it adds body and bounce. What is this magic potion? My Volume Enhancer, that's what! Made of flaxseeds, it has a lot of holding power without any of the drying properties associated with the chemically based products.

VOLUME ENHANCER

Apply once a day

1 cup flaxseeds
3 cups water

Bring the water to a boil in a glass or enamel pot. *Slowly* stir the seeds into the boiling water and reduce heat. Simmer for 10 to 20 minutes, stirring constantly, until a gel-like lotion is formed.

Strain the lotion through a fine strainer or several layers of cheesecloth into a glass jar. Discard the seeds.

Dilute with a little hot water if necessary to make it about the same consistency as the Scalp Shampoo.

Pour a small amount into the palm of your hand. Rub it into your hair and comb to distribute the lotion; or pour a small quantity into a spray bottle and squirt a little bit into your hair, then comb to distribute the gel from the roots to the ends.

Volume Enhancer works just like the expensive hair-styling products, but it is perfectly safe for both hair and scalp. It costs only pennies in comparison!

Label and store any remaining lotion in the refrigerator for up to six weeks. Take care that you don't put your fingers or comb into the solution, or you might contaminate it.

Again, I must remind you to label both the reserve supply in your refrigerator and your daily supply that you keep on your dressing table.

If you have never used a styling product, or if you are locked into that horrid hair tonic tradition, I beg you to begin using my Volume Enhancer at once! You will be amazed how light it feels on your hair and, best of all, how it doesn't become sticky when the air is humid. Other styling products seem to work like a magnet by attracting grit and grime to your hair. Not my Volume Enhancer! Your hair will feel clean at the end of the day.

13
A SHORTCUT TO HAIR GROWTH
Riquette's Magic Cut

||||||||||||||||||||||||||||||||||||||||||||||||||||||||||||||||||||||||||

A haircut, you say, has nothing to do with hair growth. Ordinarily this is correct, but when you are talking about turning peach fuzz on a balding head into healthy, thriving hair, it is quite a different story.

As I have explained, much of your hair loss can be attributed to the condition of your scalp. Waxy buildup and dead cells form a barrier that quite literally asphyxiates the roots of this baby-fine hair. Once this life-source has been smothered, your hair cannot grow.

Those silky fine hairs that you can feel when you run your fingers through your hair—that peach fuzz we have been talking about—cannot survive and grow into strong, long-lasting hair if it has to struggle to get through a wall of wax and dead cells. The root will become so weakened, because of the lack of nutrition from a healthy blood flow, that it won't be strong enough to push through the pore.

The treatments in this program, as well as thorough brushing and proper massage, will dissolve the oils and waxes blocking the scalp and will remove anything that adheres to the scalp. They will also balance the condition of the hair and scalp, normalizing the hair's acid mantle and stabilizing the flow of the sebaceous glands that keep the scalp and, in turn, the hair, pliant and lubricated.

The right haircut—one that relieves any pressure on new hair as it emerges from below the scalp—is the coup de grâce to the entire program.

I call it my Magic Cut because it works like a magic charm that helps your hair grow with ease.

Take this book with you on your next visit to your hair stylist or barber. He or she will understand exactly what to do by looking at the pictures.

Even if you do it yourself, have your hairline trimmed every three weeks. Just a tiny bit at the ends. Lift your hair with your comb and take tiny snips—even of the fuzz.

By carefully sectioning the hair and clipping the ends of each section horizontally and then resectioning so that it can be cut vertically, your stylist will be able to create "tunnels" through the underlayers of your hair. This technique provides "lift"—air space—from underneath so that your new hair will have room to grow.

In this way, any weight that might press down on the peach fuzz that we are transforming into hair will be removed.

You will find that, as you use the scalp and hair treatments and your hair begins to grow stronger and healthier than ever before, you will need to have your hair cut more often. I sug-

The hairline *must* be cut with precision and care. Every single hair must be lifted with a comb and cut. Your stylist will comb a thin layer forward and clip, then section another layer forward and clip it even with the first, repeating the process until all hair has been sectioned and cut from the front hairline to the crown.

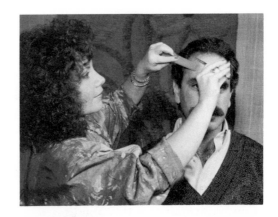

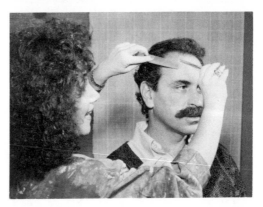

Once the horizontal layering of the top is complete, the same area must be layered and cut on an angle, vertically with the sides. Work from the front to the back on each side. Such careful distribution of the hair's volume creates a balanced, easily styled look for both men and women.

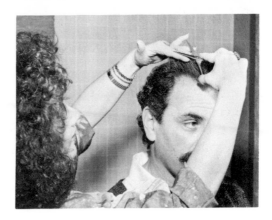

Working from the crown, your stylist will section your hair vertically in small sections. Lift hair and cut over the comb. Alternate cutting vertically with cutting horizontally until you reach the nape.

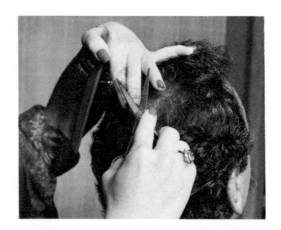

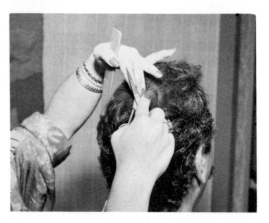

gest that the clients who come into my clinic have cuts every three or four weeks instead of every two to three months.

This is a surprise to them at first, but within the first month of the program, they understand why I say this. Their hair is growing faster than ever.

While all of the pictures illustrate the Magic Cut on men, the same cutting principles should be used for women's hair. Certainly, short hair is lighter in weight than long or even medium-length hair, but with the Magic Cut, this weight will not press down on new hair growth.

Be careful to integrate the layering from both sides and the crown so that you won't have a strong line across your head. My Magic Cut is precision haircutting at its most precise. Even fuzz like Jay has across the top of his head must be combed and clipped to prohibit damage and drying as it grows.

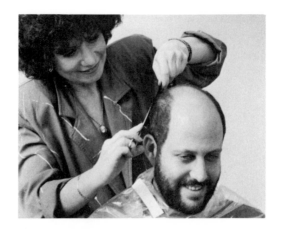

Angular cutting at the sides strengthens and shapes hair at the temples. Regular cutting will enable your hair to grow into shape. By the time you complete the twelve-week program, the styling patterns of the basic Magic Cut will be established.

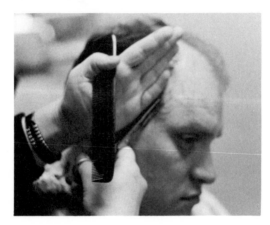

A client who has very fine but thick gray-blond hair swears by the Magic Cut because it adds volume to her relatively straight hair. As her hair is becoming gray, she has noticed that this gray hair is coarser than the blond and is slightly wavy in comparison to the super-straight ash-blond hair. The Magic Cut complements the texture of her hair, which, thanks to my regimen, is healthier than it has been since she was a little girl with cornsilk hair.

14

APPLAUSE! APPLAUSE! APPLAUSE!

Massage Makes a Difference

||||||||||||||||||||||||||||||||||||||||||||||||||||||||||||||||||||||||||||

Massage is almost as important to the success of my programs as is the application of the treatments—and it feels so good!

Few people ever rub their heads unless they have a headache. It's such a pity, but what can I expect? Many people barely touch their loved ones every day. Why should I think they might consider cuddling themselves?

I feel so strongly about the benefits of massage for the scalp, neck and face that I am going to teach you how to massage yourself and ask you to pass this technique along. You will absolutely glow, and so will your hair!

I want you to learn the proper techniques of scalp and neck massage—plus a few marvelous treats for your face—so that you can properly apply the treatments. Remember, I have asked you to *massage* the Stimulators into your scalp, and then to *massage* the Slougher Cocktail into your scalp . . . and *massage* is how you use my Scalp and Hair Shampoos!

Through my training in massage, I have learned techniques that actually increase the potency of the treatments. Scalp manipulation, as well as massage of the neck and face, stimulates blood circulation through the scalp and neck, while relaxing and soothing the nerves in your head. Still another benefit of massage is that it stimulates the muscles and activity of the various glands in the scalp, especially the sebaceous glands. Stimulation, by the way, doesn't mean that they will be producing more oil as a result of massage, but only that they will be working more efficiently. Massage renders a tight scalp more flexible and helps maintain the growth and health of the hair.

Learn to make these movements with a continuous, even motion. Use the balls of your fingertips—never the nails—and the cushions of your palms to stimulate all the activity in your scalp, your neck and even your face.

Never, ever jerk your neck about. Be gentle, not rough. Slide your fingers through your hair and concentrate all your positive energies on your scalp surface.

I asked my friend and client Ron Ronan about the benefits of massage. He should know—he's a licensed massage therapist who uses a variety of techniques to treat physical problems. Ron has seen tense, pained patients relax almost immediately after he has begun working on their heads and necks. "I think there is something neurological in the benefits of scalp massage," he says. "There are a lot of neurons—nerve centers—there. As soon as you start to work on these, people immediately begin to relax."

Ron tells me that he has had clients relax so completely on his table while he was massaging their scalp, neck and face that they have actually gone to sleep. "There is something nurturing about massage of the head and neck. . . . I have had people tell me that they have their hair shampooed and styled because they like the way it *feels*, even more than the way it looks."

Start your massage session with some simple facial exercises. They will get your circulation moving.

The kiss: Pucker your lips together in an exaggerated kiss. Hold for a count of five; relax and repeat ten times.

Chewing: Open your mouth as wide as you can. Circle your jaws in a vast chewing motion. Move slowly and deliberately, chewing and chewing for a count of twelve.

The lion: This famous yoga posture is also excellent for the face and scalp. Open your eyes as wide as you can, then open your mouth as wide as possible and stick your tongue out as far as you can, pointing the tip downward, toward your chin. Hold for a count of fifteen; relax and repeat.

Scales: A super massage technique for the face was created to ease pain of Temporomandibular Joint Syndrome (TMJ). Place your fingertips on your cheeks, feeling that recess where your upper and lower teeth mesh as you chew or talk. Move your fingers as though playing a scale on a piano, pressing as deeply and firmly as feels comfortable.

Neck rolls: Complete your warmups by slowly rotating your head from side to side five times in each direction.

Hanging: Lie on your back on a bed or table. Hang your head off the edge so that blood circulation is increased through the neck and scalp. Breathe deeply and relax. Lie there for several minutes.

Now you are ready to begin these simple scalp massage movements.

Forehead manipulation: Hold your left hand across the back of your head to steady your neck. Relax your head into your hand. Place your right hand across your forehead, stretching your thumb and forefinger across your brow line. Move your hand slowly and firmly upward to one inch past your hairline. Repeat five times.

Scalp manipulation: Place the palms of your hands firmly against your scalp above each ear. "Lift" the scalp in a circular movement, first with the hands at the side of your head, then with one hand at the top front and the other at the center back, right at the nape of your neck.

Sliding movements: With your fingertips on each side of your head, slide your fingers firmly upward. Spread your fingertips until they meet on top of your head. Repeat five times.

Hairline circles: Beginning at the hairline, place the fingers of both hands on the center of your hairline—right at your forehead. Massage around the hairline, concentrating on the areas of hair loss as you work your fingertips in a gentle circular motion. Work all the way around your hairline, including the temples, behind your ears and across the back of your neck.

Crown manipulations: Placing your fingertips at the crown, work in gentle circular movements throughout the crown. Work outward, moving forward to the temples and then back along the sides. Repeat five times.

Ear-to-ear movements: Hold your left hand across your forehead, letting your head rest in the cup made by your palm. With the fingertips of your right hand, start behind your left

Using the tips of my fingers, I massage the Stimulating Oils into the scalp. When you are working on your own scalp or that of your partner, use the tips of your fingers and rub in gentle but firm circular movements. Concentrate first on the hairline and then work into the crown and all other areas of loss, such as the part. The other benefits of massage are important not only to the success of the hair growth program but also to your personal well-being.

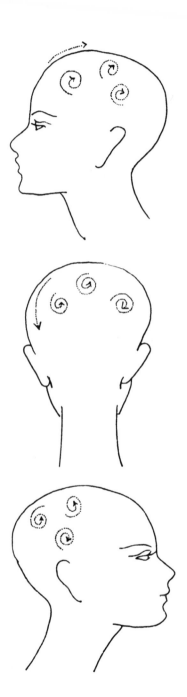

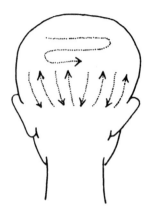

ear and make gentle but steady circular motions along the base of your skull. If you are afraid of massaging too roughly, use the heel of your palm in a rotary movement from ear to ear. Repeat twice.

Zigzags: Using your fingertips only, work in a firm up and down motion, moving from side to side. Work from the crown to the neckline and then reverse the process, zigzagging from the nape to the crown. Repeat twice.

Pulling: Gently grasp small bunches of your hair firmly with your fingertips. Pull slowly—do not yank on your hair—for a count of three and release. Repeat, pulling small bunches of hair until your entire head of hair has been tugged.

15
RADIATE SUNSHINE
Skin Care at Its Best

||||||||||||||||||||||||||||||||||||||||||||||||||||||||||||||||||||||||

Believe it or not, skin care is as much a part of my program to stop hair loss and restore hair and scalp to their healthy, shining best as any of the treatments I have taught you so far.

Men especially need to learn totally new skin-care habits. We women, for the most part, have cultivated the practice of putting on and taking off our makeup, but most men merely shower and shave, paying little if any attention to the face.

The result of this neglect is a combination of dead cells, wax and oils that build up and leave the forehead sticky and shiny.

DOS AND DON'TS OF SKIN CARE

Do apply all skin-care treatments with your finger-tips *or* pure *white* facial tissues or cotton balls. The inks in colored or printed tissues may cause skin irritations.

Don't *ever* scrub your face with terry cloth wash-cloths. The fibers of the fabric are too abrasive for your tender skin, and the laundry detergents, bleaches and softeners you use to wash them can leave a residue in the cloth that can be harmful to your skin as well.

Don't use toilet paper on your face. It is too rough and often has perfumes and deodorants in it. These products are especially harmful to facial skin.

Don't use deodorant body soaps on your face be-cause they kill *all* the bacteria—both good and bad —which destroys the acid mantle of the skin, leaving it wide open to problems.

Do use *light* circular strokes when applying any product, whether cleanser or moisturizer, toner or makeup, to your face. Work upward and out, toward the hairline.

Do massage cleansers into the forehead, as far as your hairline.

Do your skin-care program *before* you wash your hair in the morning so that you can be sure to rinse all cleansers from the hair around the hairline.

Don't ever rinse your face with hot water! It causes a condition called *couperose*—red, dilated corpuscles. Undo the damage of *couperose* by patting your face with the fingertips of both hands in a feather-light typing motion.

Do apply Toner to freshly rinsed face with clean white cotton balls, patting the Toner all over using soft upward and outward strokes. Or use a mister to spray the Toner on your face, and then distribute it with cotton balls.

Don't use alcohol or even pharmaceutically prepared witch hazel, which is a solution of witch hazel extract and alcohol, on your face, as it is too drying and can cause irritation.

Do moisturize your skin after every face-cleansing treatment. You are never too young or too old to moisturize your skin. Remember, we age not because we lose the oil in our skin but because we lose the moisture.

This shininess soon extends upward, along the hairline, weakening new hair as it grows in at the front and contributes considerably to balding.

By now you already know that wax, oil and dead cells are the "terrible trio" where hair loss is concerned. This buildup contributes to balding by making it impossible for hair to grow through the blocked pores. By ridding your forehead of this coating, you will also rid yourself of any pimples lurking under your skin.

There are three steps to my skin-care program: (1) cleansing; (2) toning; and (3) moisturizing. And they only take three minutes in the morning and three minutes at night. Finally, to absorb excess oil, you will use a clay mask once a week.

Recipes for the daily program as well as the weekly treatment are so simple that a child can make them. Unless I say otherwise, each of these recipes is for one application.

DEEP PORE MORNING CLEANSER

Apply every morning

1 tablespoon Scalp Shampoo (page 88)
1 tablespoon powdered milk, reconstituted
with 2 tablespoons water
1 teaspoon almond meal, bran or oatmeal

Mix the ingredients together in a glass bowl. Stir into a paste. Rub gently into your skin with your fingertips. Remember to include your forehead, hairline and neckline. Rinse thoroughly with cool water. Apply a light application of Toner.

NIGHTLY CLEANSER

Apply nightly

1 tablespoon Hair Shampoo (pages 88–89)
1 teaspoon wheat germ oil
or
1 teaspoon glycerine and rosewater

Mix the ingredients together in a glass bowl. Rub into your face with your fingertips. Remember your forehead, hairline and neckline. Rinse thoroughly with cool water. Apply a light application of Toner.

TONER

Apply after cleansers

3 ounces apple cider vinegar
8 ounces distilled water
1 teaspoon alum

In a bottle with a tight-fitting top, mix the ingredients together. Shake until the alum dissolves. Apply sparingly with cotton balls or use a spray bottle to spritz a mist onto your face. Distribute across your face with cotton balls.

Label container and store in the refrigerator.

Moisturizer completes each skin-care treatment. This uncomplicated recipe gives your skin that fresh, young glow.

HONEY-ALMOND MOISTURIZER

Apply twice a day

1 tablespoon honey
12 drops almond oil

In a small glass bowl, beat the honey and oil together until thoroughly mixed. Store in a small jar with a tight-fitting lid.

Dab a dot of moisturizer on each cheek, your forehead and chin. Using your fingertips, massage lightly, working upward and out toward your hairline. Take care not to get it in your hair. Use sparingly twice a day. This recipe makes approximately three applications.

Once a week, without fail, I want you to use the Mud Mask to absorb any excess oil in your face. This will help remove dead cells, keeping your face clean and healthy.

MUD MASK

Apply once a week

2 teaspoons Mud Pack (page 80)
3 tablespoons warm water

Stir the ingredients together in a glass bowl, making a light paste. Apply with your fingertips, taking care to avoid the areas around your eyes—above and below, please. Work the mask into your hairline and temples. Let dry on your face for 20 to 30 minutes, and rinse off with cool but not cold water. Pat your face dry with a clean towel.

I cannot stress enough how vital it is for you to keep your face—and especially your forehead—clean. As I tell my clients, if you wash everything but your forehead and hairline, you may as well be taking a shower with your hat on.

16
THE JEWELS IN YOUR CROWNING GLORY
Problems Particular to Women

||||||||||||||||||||||||||||||||||||||||||||||||||||||||||||||||||||

Just because we don't see many bald-headed women, it doesn't mean that women don't experience drastic hair loss. Only one woman in 20,000 may be totally bald, but there are thousands and thousands who are partially bald. Tens of thousands more have thin, weak, unmanageable hair that needs help.

We are simply more adept at the fine art of camouflaging our problems than men are. After all, we have been taught to choose our hairstyles and "do" things to our hair since we were little girls. I haven't met a woman yet who would take abnormal hair loss without putting up a fight. We jump right in and find out what alternatives are open to us, resorting to coloring, perming, wigs and hairpieces, not to mention accessories, in a pinch.

Severe hair loss in women can usually be traced to a specific physical condition—hormonal imbalance, pregnancy and childbirth, menopause or even an illness, however slight—or to the application of a product or process that damages both hair and scalp. Chemotherapy and other medical procedures can produce severe fallout, as can general ill health. After long, high fevers, for example, there will often be an increase in hair loss.

Baldness is considered a secondary sexual characteristic in men, but it is seldom inherited by women. There are, however, hereditary factors that influence some types of hair loss, especially those related to hormonal sources.

Female hair loss has become more and more evident in recent years as more and more women enter the work force and compete at the same level and pace as men. By confronting the same intensity of stress as their male co-workers and eating the same fast foods on the run, not to mention smoking and consuming alcohol at a comparable rate, women in the workplace are setting themselves up for hair loss.

More women than ever before are coming to me for hair-loss treatments. Previously, my female clients came for cuts, color, perms and conditioning; they did not need to be treated for balding.

My hair and scalp treatment program, teamed with good nutrition and thorough skin care, can produce remarkable results. One client even credits my treatments with saving her hair during a series of chemotherapy treatments.

Ilene Samson had been a skin-care client, coming to me for facials for several years. She had never consulted with me about her hair until she became ill with a debilitating thyroid imbalance. Normally an active, healthy woman with gleaming skin and hair, Ilene had become extremely sluggish and weak. That in itself was worrisome, but when her skin became dry and itchy, and her hair brittle and dull, she grew concerned. This concern turned to panic when her hair started to fall out by handfuls. "I was so depressed I would just lie on my bed and cry," she recalls.

Ilene's endocrinologist told her that hair loss was just part of her condition and that she should just buy herself a wardrobe of wigs. She refused to accept his advice, and came to me for help. "I didn't want to wear wigs," she says. "I wanted my hair back." She had heard the men in my clinic talk about how much hair they were growing, and decided to give it a try.

Ilene was ultimately diagnosed as having a severely underactive thyroid, which has been corrected by a low-dosage thyroid supplement. She has restored energy and vitality as well as beautiful, healthy hair and skin.

Now she won't let anyone but me touch her hair.

Ilene's doctor is typical. It is sad but undeniable that the medical profession understands very little about the care of the hair and scalp. Doctors usually ignore the fact that our hair reflects our overall health, and attempt to treat a specific condition, usually without results.

Dietary needs must be considered, too. Eating disorders, such as anorexia nervosa and bulimia, take a drastic toll on the body's general health and become painfully apparent in the condition of a woman's hair and scalp. Women who are constantly dieting, losing and gaining weight like a yo-yo, are neglecting the nutritional needs of their hair and cause severe damage and even loss.

Sometimes the things we do to our hair and scalp in the name of beauty are hideously harmful. We trustingly buy colors, cleansers, straighteners, perms and relaxers because we believe that these products would not be on the market if they were going to harm us. If they were dangerous, how could they be so easily available and advertised so extensively?

When Darnelia Moller came to me for a consultation, she

DeeCee's hair was most seriously damaged at the temples and above her forehead. Within a matter of weeks, dramatic regrowth had filled in the temples and across the forehead. Her hair was also thicker and healthier through the crown and in back.

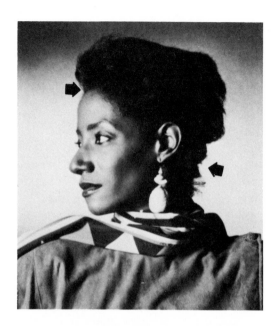

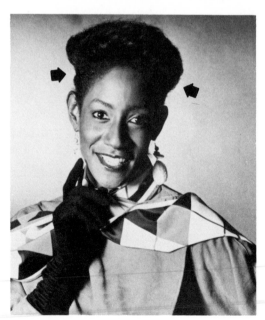

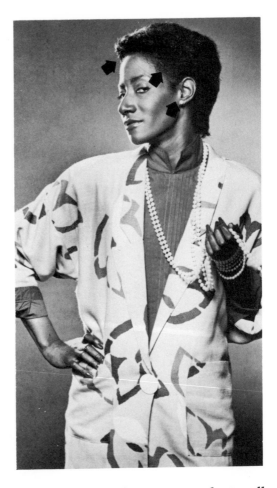

brought a giant box full to the top with hair-care products, all made to relax, straighten, process, condition and otherwise beautify black hair. She had tried them all, and now she needed some serious help!

On and off for ten years, she had used a series of hair-straightening products to relax the curl in her hair. A model who works fashion shows and in showrooms in Los Angeles, DeeCee, as I call her, felt that she had more styling versatility with looser, softer curl about her face and through her crown.

TIPS FOR SAFE HAIR STYLING

Don't brush hair when it's wet. If you do, the hair will break. Comb wet hair gently with a smooth-toothed comb. The teeth of the comb should have no rough, sharp edges.

Don't blow-dry your hair at the hottest temperature. Take a few more minutes and use a lower temperature. Even better, allow your hair to dry naturally whenever possible.

If you use rollers, set your hair on large ones without tension. Rolling the hair too tightly will put stress on the roots, causing breakage and loss. Use end papers if you use rollers. Curling irons or electric rollers should be used at a low temperature. Hot curling tools can cause breakage and drying and can also overstimulate the sebaceous glands in the scalp. This means your scalp will be too oily!

Don't go out in the sun without protecting your hair with a hat. And never sunbathe without washing the salty sea water or chemical-filled pool water from your hair and then putting on a hat or scarf. Before swimming, rinse out styling gels, mousses and sprays (which are full of alcohol and other chemicals). Protect your hair and scalp by rubbing Basic Stimulator (page 72) into your scalp and the ends of your hair before going swimming or spending time in the sun.

In cold weather, protect your hair with a hat or scarf. Frigid temperatures can be as brutal on your hair as hot weather and pollution!

Barely fourteen weeks after she had been forced to crop her shoulder-length, relaxed hair because it had been severely damaged by ten years of chemical processing, DeeCee was back on the runway, modeling for an American Lung Association benefit.

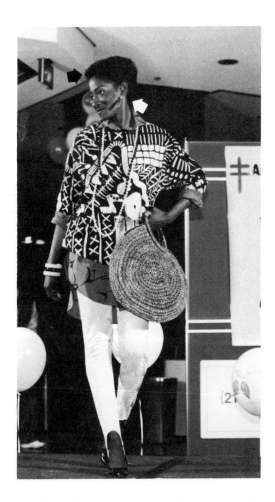

After a while, her hair could no longer tolerate the chemicals and the "heat perms," and it began to break off and fall out.

By the time DeeCee came to me, she had to have what was left of her shoulder-length hair cropped close to her head. She wore hats and wigs whenever she left her house until her sensitive scalp and thin, porous hair were well on their way to recovery.

During this time, when her hair was at its worst, DeeCee

would not allow herself to be photographed unless she was draped in scarves or wore a head-covering hat of some sort. She couldn't. Models with thin, brittle, dry, damaged hair don't get a lot of work!

Hair that is chemically treated, for whatever reason, has had its texture altered. It is more susceptible to breakage and loss than untreated hair.

Regardless of the cause and the hair type, treatment for damaged, thinning hair is the same for a woman as for a man. Look back at the basic program and start this very minute on your way to creating a luxurious, lovely head of healthy hair.

17

YOU'RE NEVER TOO YOUNG TO TAKE CARE OF YOUR HAIR

Riquette's Hair Preservation Program for Children Through Age Twelve

||||||||||||||||||||||||||||||||||||||||||||||||||||||||||||||||||||||||||

Just as you are never too old to start caring for your hair and scalp, you're never too young to take care of yourself—especially if you want a lifetime of healthy, shining hair.

When we are born, we have soft, wispy fuzz all over our heads. As we mature, this baby fuzz generally is replaced by darker hair that is thicker and coarser. By the time a child reaches adolescence, he or she has hair with all the qualities of adult hair. And, more than likely, the child has a mountain of bad habits where hair and skin are concerned! After all, they copy their parents.

It is very important for young people—boys especially—to learn to care for their hair. Otherwise, there is a very good possibility that they will be bald in adulthood. Balding is a secondary sexual trait in males, and unless steps are taken to prevent hair loss by every means possible—hair and scalp care as well as diet and nutrition—these hormonal and hereditary factors will win out. Currently, I am treating a young man of sixteen for hair loss in my clinic. I have seen balding begin even younger. However, if you start your children on this program before they enter adolescence—when they are nine or ten—and instill the habit of proper hair care in children from the time of their first haircut, I promise you that they will never have a problem with hair loss!

When my nephews and nieces were mere babies, I started cutting and caring for their hair. My sister taught them how to wash and care for their hair and skin properly when they were very small, so that now, as teenagers and young adults, they have shining, healthy hair and no skin problems whatsoever. This is no accident. Acne and other skin problems, not to mention dry, fragile hair, run in our family.

Unfortunately, most young people are not so lucky. Young boys, especially, hate showers and hate to wash their hair. They go swimming or surfing and, without so much as a spray of a shower, head for the park for baseball practice. Or they stay out in the cold, skiing and skating and sledding as long as there's a speck of light in the sky. As much fun as this can be, it can be devastating to the hair. Extreme weather conditions, hot or cold, as well as the chemicals of the pool, for instance, combine with the fact that your son has not actually washed his hair with shampoo to remove excess oils and everything else that might be stuck to it. The result is an environment conducive to massive hair loss.

We must teach our children when they are small about how to care for their hair, scalp and skin so that they will never, ever have problems.

Your child will use the same products that you do—the

RIQUETTE'S HAIR PRESERVATION PROGRAM
for Children Through Age Twelve

DAILY
  Brush hair
  Wash hair and brush
    Scalp Shampoo (page 88)
    Hair Shampoo (page 88)
  Rinse with tepid water
  Protective Sealing Lotion (page 92)
  Volume Enhancer (pages 96–97)

WEEKLY
  Protein Pack (page 84)
    (Apply to damp hair)
  Wash hair and brush
    Scalp Shampoo
    Hair Shampoo
  Rinse with tepid water
  Protective Sealing Lotion
  Volume Enhancer

AFTER SWIMMING AND PLAYING SPORTS
  Wash hair
    Hair Shampoo
  Rinse with tepid water
  Protective Sealing Lotion
  Volume Enhancer

same shampoos, Protective Sealing Lotion and Volume Enhancer. Once a week your child will use the Protein Pack, just as you do, so you can make a family project of hair care.

Even if your child's father, his grandfathers and all of his uncles on both sides of the family are bald, your child doesn't have to be bald. And, just as your son will avert dramatic hair loss, your daughter will get a head start toward a magnificent mane of shining hair.

TEACHING YOUR CHILDREN GOOD HAIR-CARE HABITS

Make daily bathtime and hair-washing fun. Not a game, but enjoyable. Even small children should be able to wash their hair every day. We adults have learned to do it, and we take care that our infants are washed every day, so why do we let the daily wash cycle pass, once our young ones become the least bit independent and insist upon bathing themselves?

Although the Hair and Scalp Shampoo recipes on pages 88–89 are completely safe for a child's hair and scalp, you may find "tearless" baby shampoo helpful when teaching your children to wash their own heads. Once they have the knack of hair washing, switch to the products I have created for this program.

Teach your children how to brush and comb their hair, and then give them the right tools to use so that they don't scratch their scalps and break their hair. *Give each child his or her* own *brush and comb*. Like toothbrushes, they are not to be shared. Use natural-bristle brushes because they will not damage the hair.

Show your children how to brush their hair, using firm but gentle strokes without pulling. Brushing *does* keep hair and scalp healthy, provided it's done correctly.

Never let your child brush wet hair. Instead, teach them to comb out tangles with a wide-tooth comb.

Children should also be taught to wash their brushes and combs daily, as part of their daily hair-washing ritual.

Don't ever comb your child's hair from above so that you make a long part from the crown in the back to the forehead in front. This only pulls hair in an unnatural direction and weakens it from the root. This sets a pattern for balding later on. Instead, start your child's part from the front hairline, combing hair back just a bit—not beyond the ear—and let hair fall naturally. Become aware of your child's natural part. If at all possible, let that be the guide for where you make the part. For most people, this natural part falls on the left or in the center, with relatively few people having natural parts on the right.

After washing, blot out excess water with a terry cloth towel, then rub the hair almost dry. Comb gently to remove tangles, working them out from the ends to the roots; this avoids pulling hair out by the roots. Whenever possible, let hair dry naturally. Don't blow-dry your child's hair at a high temperature because this can burn both hair and scalp.

Have your child's hair cut regularly. As a general rule, the shorter you keep your hair when you are young, the better off you will be as an adult. This, however, is not always practical. Styles, as we all know, don't always suit what is truly best for us.

Have your child's hair professionally trimmed at the ends every four to six weeks.

18
RIQUETTE'S CUISINE DE BEAUTÉ
Make Your Own Private Label Cosmetics

||||||||||||||||||||||||||||||||||||||||||||||||||||||||||||||||||||||||||||||||||

As promised, I will tell you how to add variety and spice to your hair, scalp and skin care repertoire.

In my basic Hair Rejuvenation Program, I have given you recipes that use a very select group of powerful natural ingredients known through the ages for their restorative, healing properties.

Believe me, narrowing down my choice and deciding which of the recipes in my arsenal of treatments would be most effective, simplest to prepare, and easiest to use, proved to be a very difficult task for me. I wanted to share with you every single one of the treatments and products I have in my recipe file!

When I came to my senses, I decided I would give you the basic program that will provide you with results, and then supplement it with the following "graduate course" in the use of herbs, with recipes that employ many other wonderful gifts of nature. Even this barely scratches the surface of available compounds!

Do not use these recipes during the first twelve weeks of treatments. Stick to the original plan *without fail*, and without any additions and changes. You have a lifetime ahead of you to play with new, natural treatments.

Here I will give you alternative treatments that retard balding and encourage new growth. I have also included some new treatments that you can add to your routine—natural colors, for example, that you might want to use to darken your new hair as it begins to grow, making it more visible. These natural coloring rinses are the *only* supplementary treatments that you have my permission to use right now. They are completely safe and will enhance your new hair as it grows.

Before I give you the recipes, I want to share the following list of nature's gifts for your hair and skin. I have broken these herbs, flowers, roots and other organic botanical treasures down by use—conditioners, dandruff treatments, and treatments for oiliness or dryness, for example. It gives you an idea of why I had such difficulty selecting the ingredients for my basic program!

After you have completed the twelve-week treatment program, you have my permission to mix and match ingredients in the recipes. For example, you might try adding nettles to the infusion used in your Scalp Shampoo, or substitute a decoction of quassia chips for the boiling water that moistens the fuller's earth and henna for the weekly Mud Pack.

Brunettes might want to add cloves, coffee or raspberry to

the infusion used to make the Protective Sealing Lotion; cowslip, marigolds or yarrow could add life to blond or golden hair.

NATURAL HAIR-CARE INGREDIENTS

Conditioners

Basil oil
Cherry bark
Lavender oil
Nettle and cherry bark (infusion)

Ragwort
Rosemary (leaves and oil)

Dandruff

Artichoke
Bergamot vinegar
Chamomile
Juniper leaves
Lemongrass
Lemon juice
Lemon oil

Mint vinegar
Nettle
Orange peel
Quassia chips
Rosemary
Soap root
Willow

Dryness

Acacia
Chamomile
Clover
Comfrey root

Cowslip
Elder
Orange flower
Peach flower

General care

Avocado oil
Almond oil
Beets
Blackcurrant
Brewer's yeast
Burdock root
Dandelion
Dulse
Elder
Jaborandi
Kelp
Lemongrass
Lemon oil

Maidenhair fern
Nettle
Olive oil
Onion juice
Parsley
Pineapple juice
Rosemary
Southernwood
Vinegar (apple cider or
   white, depending upon
   hair color)
Walnut oil
Yarrow

Growth (to stimulate growth)

American bearsfoot
Basil oil
Jaborandi
Lady's smock
Lavender oil

Lemon oil
Nettle
Onion juice
Rosemary leaves
Southernwood

Loss (to dislodge oils)

Basil oil
Gobernadora
Lavender oil
Nettle

Peach
Rosemary (leaves and oil)
Sage and borax
Southernwood

Oiliness

Bergamot
Lemongrass
Lemon peel
Orris root
Peppermint oil

Quassia chips
Rosebuds
White willow bark
Witch hazel bark

Scalp (for irritated, sensitive scalps)

Birch bark
Horsetail
Rosemary (oil and leaves)

Speedwell
Yarrow

Shine

Chamomile
Lemon peel
Maidenhair fern
Marigold

Nettle
Raspberry
Rosemary
Sage

Split Ends

Almond oil
Basil oil
Lavender oil
Nutmeg oil

Olive oil
Peanut oil
Rosemary oil
Walnut oil

NATURAL HAIR COLORINGS

Make decoctions or infusions of these natural products, then use these liquids to rinse color into your hair. You won't see the immediate results associated with chemical coloring processes but, instead, will see gradual color that intensifies with continued use.

Blond or Light

Chamomile
Comfrey root
Cowslip flowers
Elder flowers
Grapefruit peel
Lemon juice
Lemon peel

Marigold flowers
Mullein (yellow)
Orange peel
Orris root
White vinegar
White willow bark
Yarrow

Golden Blond

Bedstraw
Beets
Chamomile

Henna
Marigold flowers

Brown or Reddish Brown

Beets
Cinnamon
Cloves
Coffee

Henna
Indigo
Sage

Brunette

Apple cider vinegar
Bergamot
Cloves
Coffee
Henna
Jaborandi
Nettle

Quassia chips
Raspberries
Rosemary
Sage
Southernwood
Thyme

NATURAL SKIN-CARE INGREDIENTS

Acne

Cantaloupe
Golden seal
Honey
Lavender

Mango
Papaya
Sea salt
White willow bark

Blackheads

Buttermilk
Honey

Pansy
Violet

Complexion

Almond milk
Caraway
Coriander
Jamaica flowers

Parsley
Rosewater
Yogurt

Dry Skin

Aloe vera	Milk
Anise	Mint
Apple	Oatmeal
Chamomile	Olive oil
Caraway	Orange blossom
Clover	Orange peel
Comfrey (leaves and	Orris root
roots)	Pansy
Cowslip	Parsley
Dandelion	Peach
Fennel	Strawberry
Honeydew	Violet
Licorice	Yarrow

Emollients

Almond oil	Lecithin
Aloe vera	Malva flowers
Apricot oil	Marshmallow root
Cocoa butter	Mint
Comfrey	Oatmeal
Flax	Orange flowers
Flaxseed oil	Quince seeds
Glycerine	Slippery elm
Honey	Wheat germ oil
Lanolin	

Exfoliants

Catsfoot	Pineapple
Lemon juice	Tomato
Papaya	

Normal Skin

All fruits
All grains
All vegetables
Avocado

Banana
Leek
Peach

Oily Skin

Anise
Apricot
Caraway
Cucumber
Dandelion
Dulse
Fennel
Lavender

Lemon (juice, oil and
  peel)
Lemongrass
Licorice
Papaya
Rose
Witch hazel

Pimples

Almond meal
Comfrey
Milk
Oatmeal

Papaya
Peppermint
Yogurt

Pores

Almond meal
Buttermilk
Camphor (oil)
Coltsfoot
Comfrey
Egg white

Elder flower
Honey
Lavender
Oatmeal
Papaya
Parsley

Pores *(continued)*

Peach
Pennyroyal
Peppermint
Sandalwood

Strawberry
Vinegar
White willow bark

Scaling

Avocado
Papaya
Salt

Sensitive or Irritated Skin

Aloe vera
Avocado
Birch bark
Comfrey
Cranberry
Egg (inner skin, white)
Elder
Figwort
Fuchsia

Lavender
Marigold
Rose
Sassafras
Sorrel
Tansy
Walnut (leaves, bark)
Yarrow

Tone

Bay
Chamomile
Celery
Honey

Orange blossoms
Salt
Sandalwood
Vetivert

If you don't think you're ready to experiment on your own, you might be interested in some of the following suggestions:

ADDITIONAL STIMULATORS

The Basic Stimulator and the Super Stimulator that get to the root of your hair in the basic program use the most stimulating oils available. However, after six or eight months, you may decide your scalp needs a change of pace. The two Rejuvenating Stimulators that follow may be just what you're looking for to get yourself back on track. Use only for two weeks, then return to the original recipes.

REJUVENATING STIMULATOR I

Use 10 drops of each of the following essential oils:

> *arnica*
> *avocado*
> *basil*
> *comfrey*
> *eucalyptus*
> *fennel*
> *juniper*
> *lavender*
> *lemon peel*
> *rosemary*
> *savory*

Mix the oils together in an amber glass bottle with a secure dropper top. Use as a substitute for the Super Stimulator.

REJUVENATING STIMULATOR II

Use 10 drops of each of the following essential oils:

> *cypress*
> *eucalyptus*
> *pine needle*

Mix the oils together in an amber glass bottle with a glass dropper top. Use as a substitute for the Super Stimulator.

Should your scalp become sensitive or irritated for some reason, this Antiseptic Stimulator will facilitate healing.

ANTISEPTIC STIMULATOR

> *White iodine (10% solution)*

Pour a small amount of the iodine into a small glass bowl. Section dry hair and apply white iodine to the scalp with a clean triangular makeup sponge. Cover head with a hot towel for 15 to 20 minutes. Rinse with tepid water. (*Note*: Do not use hot towels on any other stimulating treatment.)

HEALTHY HAIR STIMULATOR

> *2 ounces rosemary oil*
> *2 ounces fresh lemon juice*

Mix the ingredients together in an amber bottle with a secure top. Use half for one treatment. Pour into a glass bowl and apply to scalp with your fingertips. Store in the refrigerator to prevent deterioration of juice. Must be used within one week.

WATER-ACTIVATED STIMULATOR

Use 5 drops of each of the following essential oils:

> *cinnamon*
> *cypress*
> *lavender*
> *pine*
> *sandalwood*
> *savory*
>
> *⅛ teaspoon finely powdered thyme*
> *⅛ teaspoon finely powdered oregano*

Combine the essential oils in a small glass bowl. Add thyme and oregano. Apply mixture to your scalp with your fingertips. Apply a bit of water and rub to activate oils. Work water into your hair with your fingertips, using more and more water until most of the oils have been massaged into the scalp. Use as a substitute for the Super Stimulator.

ANOTHER ROUND OF SLOUGHERS

My Slougher Cocktail is my trademark treatment, but I do know of other compounds that produce very acceptable results. Here are some variations on the theme that you may try, *only* after you have completed the twelve-week program.

SIMPLE SLOUGHER

> *10 aspirin tablets*
> *3 tablespoons liquid castile soap*

With a mortar and pestle, crush aspirins into a powder and put in a glass bowl. Adding a little castile soap at a time, make into a thick paste. Apply to the scalp with a soft toothbrush, working the scalp one section at a time.

SALT SLOUGHER
(to heal and cleanse the scalp)

1 tablespoon table salt
1 tablespoon coarsely ground sea salt
1 teaspoon pure liquid castile soap (as needed for paste)

In a glass bowl, work the two kinds of salt and the soap into a thick paste. Section hair and brush into scalp with a soft toothbrush. Massage with your fingertips.

GLYCERINE AND BORAX SLOUGHER

1 teaspoon borax (sodium tetraborate, a gentle, natural cleanser and astringent)
2 teaspoons glycerine
4 ounces warm water

In a glass bowl, stir borax and glycerine together. Slowly add water to make a loose paste. Apply to scalp with a toothbrush and work in small sections until entire head is covered.

FRESH FRUIT SLOUGHER

1 medium papaya, peeled and cubed
or
1 cup fresh *pineapple, peeled and cubed*
1 to 3 tablespoons liquid castile soap

Puree fruit in a blender, or mash completely with a fork in a glass bowl. Slowly stir soap into the fruit (the more fruit you have, the more soap you need). Apply to dry scalp with a soft toothbrush. The enzymes from the fruit help remove buildup of dry, dead skin and wax.

SLOUGHER FOR DAMAGED
OR TENDER SCALP

1 small can evaporated milk

Pour milk into a small bowl. Using either an eye dropper or cotton balls, apply a little at a time to the scalp after sectioning hair. Do *not* use a toothbrush, no matter how soft yours is. Instead, massage the milk into your scalp with your fingertips.

Your scalp may be sensitive and tender, but it still needs this treatment to deter buildup. Use only when your scalp is broken out or sensitive. If this condition continues for more than two weeks, see a doctor.

MORE DIAMONDS IN THE ROUGH: ADDITIONAL MUD PACKS

Not every mud pack is made of mud.

These special treatments are designed to balance the activity of your hair and scalp while absorbing oils on the scalp.

HEALING MUD PACK
(for sensitive scalps)

1 ounce powdered cinnamon
1 ounce powdered rosemary
1 ounce powdered geranium leaves
1 ounce powdered savory
1 ounce powdered basil
1 ounce powdered oregano
1 ounce powdered cloves

Mix powdered herbs in a jar with a tight-fitting lid. Shake thoroughly.

Put ½ cup powder mixture in a glass bowl, and add enough warm water to make a thick paste. Apply with a pastry brush; let dry thoroughly.

QUICKIE MUD PACK

white of 1 large egg

Whip egg white until fluffy. Apply to dry scalp with pastry brush. Leave on for 15 minutes.

GREEN MUD

The following green vegetables, alone or in equal amounts in any combination (a sample mixture might be a handful of spinach, a bunch of parsley and a small zucchini, chopped):

> *broccoli*
> *cucumber*
> *parsley*
> *spinach*
> *turnip greens*
> *zucchini*
> *or any other green vegetables*

Steam the vegetables in ½ cup of water. When tender, puree in the blender, using the water from steaming to moisten if necessary to form a paste. Let cool before applying to scalp with a pastry brush.

POWDER PACK

1 ounce powdered juniper berries
1 ounce powdered sage
1 ounce powdered cloves
1 ounce powdered peppermint leaves
1 ounce powdered lemon peel
1 ounce powdered eucalyptus leaves
1 ounce powdered valerian root

Put powdered herbs into a glass jar that can be tightly sealed. Shake to mix.

In a glass bowl, mix ½ cup herbal powder mixture with hot water, adding water a teaspoon at a time, to work into a thick paste. Section hair and brush into scalp until completely covered. Leave on until completely dry, 20 to 30 minutes.

ADDITIONAL PROTEIN PACKS

With these simple protein packs to strengthen the shaft of your hair, you'll be as powerful as Samson—before Delilah, of course.

BASIC PROTEIN PACK FOR DARK HAIR

2 tablespoons blackstrap molasses

Apply to clean, damp hair with a pastry brush. Comb through hair. Leave on for 1 hour. Rinse with Protective Sealing Lotion or vinegar diluted in water until water runs clear.

Because the molasses may darken the hair, I do not recommend this very powerful Protein Pack for blond or gray hair.

FRUIT PACK

¼ cup bone marrow (Ask your butcher to split several beef bones. Boil bones in enough water to cover until the marrow slips out of the cut bone. Let cool before using.)
1 egg yolk
½ cup fruit (avocado, melon, etc.)
1 tablespoon vegetable oil

In a glass bowl, stir ingredients together with a fork to make a loose paste.

Apply to your hair and scalp with a pastry brush. Cover with a plastic shower cap for 30 minutes.

MOISTURIZING PROTEIN PACK

1 tablespoon honey
2 egg yolks

Mix honey and egg yolks together in a glass bowl. Apply with a pastry brush and comb through hair. Leave on hair for 20 minutes. Rinse with *cool* water.

LECITHIN PROTEIN PACK

3 ounces protein powder
3 ounces soy lecithin
2 ounces cider vinegar

In a glass bowl, stir the ingredients together to make a loose paste. Apply to hair and scalp with pastry brush and leave on for 20 minutes. Rinse with warm water.

DRY SCALP PACK

2 tablespoons mayonnaise
1 tablespoon soy sauce

In a glass bowl, stir mayonnaise and soy sauce together until completely mixed. Brush into ends of hair only. Leave on for 10 minutes. Rinse.

SHAMPOOS GALORE

These natural cleansing products will add variety to your hair-care routine. Again, I am giving you a selection of scalp shampoos and hair shampoos.

Please keep up the plan that I have given you, substituting one scalp shampoo for another and one hair shampoo for another, should you wish to expand your repertoire.

EMERGENCY DRY SHAMPOO

1 to 3 tablespoons corn meal, fuller's earth or corn starch

Wrap cheesecloth or gauze (or a cotton sweatsock in a *real* emergency) around a dry hairbrush.

Work the powder of your choice into *dry* hair and then brush it out.

This is ideal for someone who is sick or bedridden, or for those unexpected dates after a long, hard day, when you don't have time to *really* wash your hair.

SIMPLE SCALP SHAMPOO

2 egg whites
¼ cup liquid castile soap

Beat egg whites lightly, until they form light peaks. Fold in liquid castile soap. Makes a creamy astringent scalp shampoo. Store excess in the refrigerator for up to 2 weeks.

DRY SCALP SHAMPOO

10 drops pine oil
10 drops cypress oil
10 drops eucalyptus oil
10 drops naiouli
2 cups liquid castile soap

Mix the ingredients together in a bottle with a tight-fitting lid. Slowly shake or stir until thoroughly blended. Use 1 teaspoon per washing as a scalp shampoo.

STIMULATING SCALP SHAMPOO

3 ounces rosemary leaves
1 heaping teaspoon baking soda
1 quart boiling water

In a glass container with a tight lid, mix ingredients together. Cover and set aside overnight.

Add:
4 ounces rum

Strain and mix 1 cup of this infusion with 1 cup liquid castile soap.

Store remaining infusion in the refrigerator. Can be used as a stimulating rinse or saved for future use in shampoo.

NORMAL HAIR SHAMPOO

2 tablespoons thyme
2 tablespoons rosemary
2 tablespoons sage
2 tablespoons parsley
1 quart plus ½ cup boiling water
2 ounces liquid castile soap

Soak herbs in water for 2 hours. Strain and discard herbs. Slowly add castile soap to the herbal infusion and bring to a slow boil for 5 minutes. Allow to cool before using. Use 1 teaspoon per washing.

DRY HAIR SHAMPOO

2 tablespoons acacia
2 tablespoons clover
2 tablespoons lemongrass
1 quart plus ½ cup boiling water
2 ounces liquid castile soap
½ avocado, mashed

Infuse herbs for 2 hours in boiling water. Strain and discard herbs. Add liquid castile soap to water and return to a slow boil for 5 minutes. Puree avocado and stir into mixture until smooth. Allow to cool before using. Use 1 teaspoon per washing.

SHAMPOO FOR DRY, DAMAGED
OR TREATED HAIR

2 cups liquid castile soap
½ cup honey
¼ cup olive oil
1 teaspoon vitamin B oil

In a glass jar with a tight lid, combine all ingredients, stirring gently to blend.

Use 1 teaspoon per washing.

Rinse with tepid water and follow with Protective Sealing Lotion or Finishing Rinse.

ADDITIONAL PROTECTIVE
SEALING LOTIONS

Finishing rinses or sealing lotions are very possibly the most exciting way we can use herbs and other botanical ingredients to benefit our hair.

We can add color, treat dandruff, add body—just about everything! The most important function, of course, is the protection of the hair shaft.

If you're going for the gold, so to speak, and are using herbal hair colors, don't be shocked by the results of your first application. Unlike chemical color processes, herbal color is cumulative. It builds up over several applications, so don't expect golden or copper highlights the first time you use a chamomile or marigold rinse!

SIMPLE SEALING LOTION

1 cup cider vinegar
1 gallon warm water

Mix and pour through your hair.

FINISHING RINSE FOR DARK HAIR

Steep used coffee grounds in a gallon of warm water overnight. Strain and use liquid to rinse hair. Acids in the coffee seal the hair shaft, while the coffee adds warm tones.

TEA RINSE

Save used tea bags—any kind—and steep overnight in warm water. Use liquid as a sealing rinse to restore the acid mantle of the hair and scalp. The kind of tea you use determines the color of the highlights you create. Use the Natural Hair Colorings herbal chart (pages 136–137) as a reference when selecting your teas: chamomile tea imparts gold highlights, hibiscus tea gives red highlights, etc.

BLOND SEALING LOTION

1 tablespoon chamomile
1 tablespoon marigold
1 tablespoon acacia
1 quart warm water

Steep herbs until the infusion is golden. Pour through hair as a final rinse.

LEMON RINSE
(for blond and brown hair)

Juice of 1 lemon
1 quart water

In a glass bowl, strain lemon juice into warm water and pour through hair. Lemon restores the acid balance of hair and scalp, providing a sealing action, while adding gold and yellow highlights. Do not use this rinse before going out in the sun without drying your hair first, or you'll have orange hair instead of gold.

SEALING LOTION FOR BROWN HAIR

1 tablespoon rosemary
1 tablespoon sage
1 tablespoon cloves
1 tablespoon quassia chips
1 gallon water

Infuse herbs in water for at least 10 minutes. Strain and discard herbs. Pour liquid through hair for rich brown highlights.

HENNA RINSE

1 tablespoon neutral henna
1 gallon warm water

Dissolve Henna in warm water. Pour through hair. Should you want to add highlights, use colored henna. Color will build up over time.

ENHANCED VOLUME ENHANCERS

Many natural products can be safely used as styling aids for your hair.

Why use something that could be damaging to your hair—containing alcohol and other chemicals—when these natural, safe products are so easy to use?

BEER LOTION

1 can beer, any brand

Pour beer into a jar with a tight lid. Use flat beer undiluted as a styling lotion.

GEL LOTION

1 envelope unflavored gelatin
2 cups warm water

Dissolve gelatin in water. Comb through hair to add volume. Can dilute further and apply with a spray bottle.

COLORED GEL LOTION

1 tablespoon gelatin dessert, any color
1 cup warm water

Select the color of your gelatin according to the color of your hair and the highlights you want to add. Dissolve in warm water and use as a styling lotion. Comb through hair and style.

STIFFENING LOTION

½ cup cane sugar
1 cup boiling water

Dissolve sugar in boiling water, stirring until completely dissolved. Add water a tablespoon at a time if needed. Comb into hair for a stiff, firm hold.

WEIGHTS AND MEASUREMENTS

||||||||||||||||||||||||||||||||||||||||||||||||||||||||||||||||||||||||||

When preparing the recipes that will restore life to your hair, you'll need to know some simple measurements. Keep this chart handy for ready reference.

GRAIN	DRY	FLUID
15 grains	= ¼ teaspoon	= 15 drops
60 grains	= 1 teaspoon	= 60 drops

DRAM		
1 dram	= 1 teaspoon	= 1 teaspoon or 1 fluid dram

TEASPOON/TABLESPOON		
1 teaspoon	= ⅓ tablespoon	= 60 drops
1 tablespoon	= 3 teaspoons or ½ ounce	= ½ fluid ounce
2 tablespoons	= 28 grams or 1 ounce	= 1 fluid ounce
4 tablespoons	= ¼ cup	= 2 fluid ounces
16 tablespoons	= 1 cup or 8 ounces	= ½ pint or 8 fluid ounces

OUNCE		
1 ounce	= 28 grams	
16 ounces	= 2 cups or 1 pint	= 128 fluid drams
32 ounces	= 1¾ pounds or 4 cups	= 32 fluid ounces or 2 pints or 1 quart
1 kilogram	= 2 pounds 3 ounces	= 1 quart
1 liter		= 1 quart plus ½ cup
1 milliliter		= .270 fluid drams
1 gallon		= 3.785 liters

SOURCE GUIDE

||||||||||||||||||||||||||||||||||||||||||||||||||||||||||||||||||||||||||||||

Aphrodisia Products, Inc.
282 Bleecker Street
New York, NY 10014
(212) 989–6440

> This Greenwich Village shop stocks just about everything having to do with herbs, including books, teas, oils, and even cosmetics. They do not take telephone orders, but do an extensive mail-order business. Send $1 for catalogue.

Caswell-Massey Co., Ltd.
Catalogue Division
111 Eighth Avenue
New York, NY 10011
(212) 620–0900

> With wonderful stores in sixteen states and Washington, D.C., and in Canada, this delightful company offers basic ingredients for homemade cosmetics. Telephone orders may be placed weekdays between 9:00 A.M. and 7:00 P.M. (EST), and Saturdays between 10:00 A.M. and 5:00 P.M. Established in 1752, Caswell-Massey is the oldest chemist and perfumer in America. Their catalogue reflects this historic tradition. Caswell-Massey often has in stock that hard-to-find oil of basil, as well as pure castile bars with no additives.

Haussman's Pharmacy
Sixth and Girard Avenue
Philadelphia, PA 19127
(215) 627–2143

> This incredible resource of herbal mixtures, ingredients and herbs takes both telephone and mail orders. Write for their catalogue.

Herb Products Company
(Living Herbs, Inc.)
11012 Magnolia Boulevard
North Hollywood, CA 91601
(213) 877–3104 or
(818) 984–3141

> The owner and staff here are *very* helpful and are willing to answer any questions you might have. Write for their price list (twenty-five cents) today! They have essential oils and dried herbs of every sort. A minimum one-ounce order is required for oils, and a minimum four-ounce order for herbs, which are sold in four-ounce increments.

Indiana Botanic Gardens, Inc.
626 177th Street
Hammond, IN 46325
(219) 931–2480

> A find for mail-order shoppers, this excellent herb store sells all basic cosmetic ingredients, including castile soap powder for shampoo. Write for their catalogue, which has the full list of herbs and herbal products. You can also place phone orders if you call on weekdays.

Kiehl Pharmacy
109 Third Avenue
New York, NY 10003
(212) 465–3400

> *The* place for pure essential oils, Kiehl carries a large stock of cosmetic herbs. They don't offer a mail-order catalogue, but will take telephone orders with a major credit card. Hours are 10:00 A.M. to 6:00 P.M. (EST) weekdays, 10:00 A.M. to 4:30 P.M. Saturdays.

Mayway Trading Co.
622 Broadway
San Francisco, CA 94133
(415) 433–3765

> This bustling but friendly company carries a full line of herbs, selling both retail and wholesale and by mail or telephone. Write for a catalogue.

Penn Herb Company
603 North Second Street
Philadelphia, PA 19123
(215) 925–3336

> The Penn Herb catalogue is legendary! It is an absolute must for anyone who wants to become a gourmet chef of health and beauty. Penn Herb has just about everything you will need to become seriously involved in herbal skin and hair care.

INDEX